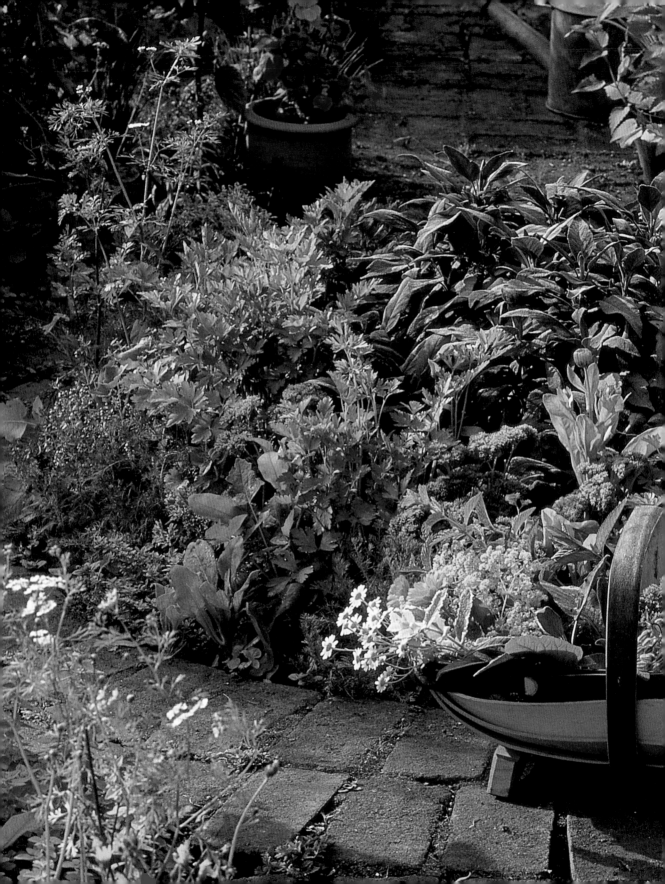

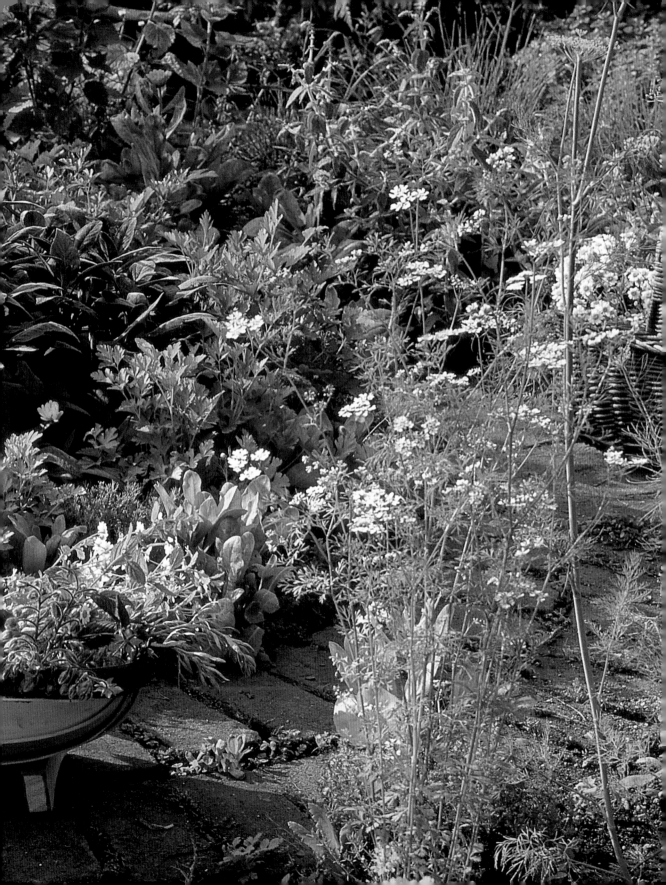

THE MEDICINAL GARDEN

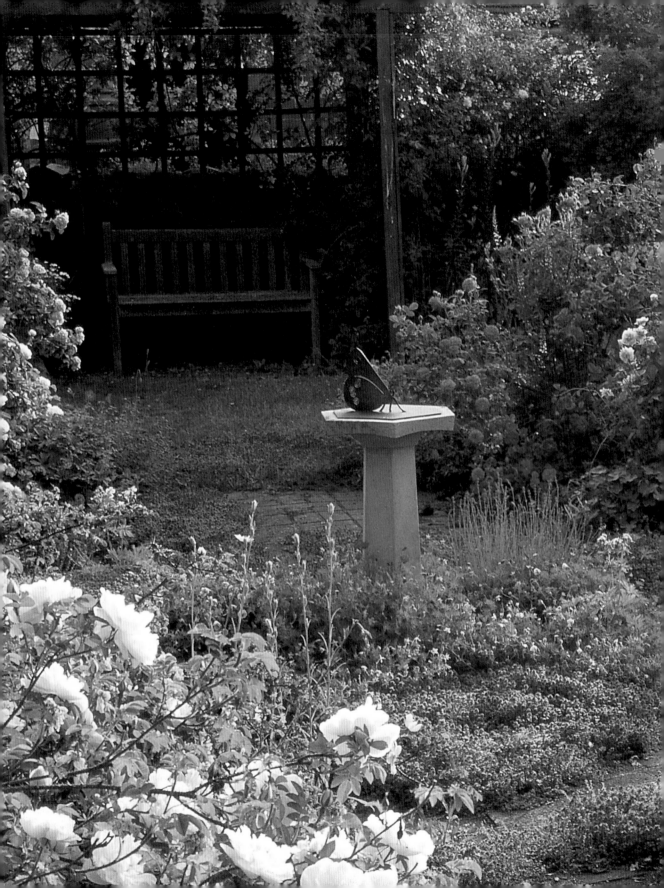

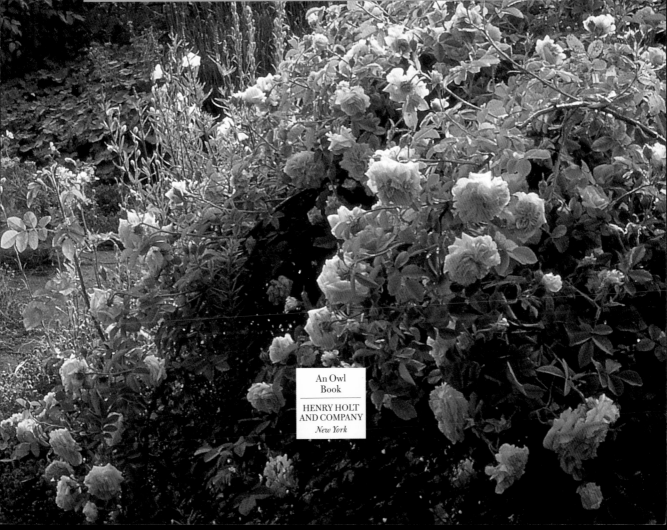

The Medicinal Garden

How to Grow and Use
Your Own Medicinal Herbs

ANNE McINTYRE

An Owl
Book

HENRY HOLT
AND COMPANY
New York

Henry Holt and Company, Inc.
Publishers since 1866
115 West 18th Street
New York, New York 10011

Henry Holt ® is a registered trademark
of Henry Holt and Company, Inc.

Published in Canada by Fitzhenry & Whiteside Ltd.,
195 Allstate Parkway, Markham, Ontario L3R 4T8

First published in 1997 by Judy Piatkus (Publishers) Ltd.
under the title *The Apothecary's Garden*.
Conceived and produced by Breslich & Foss Ltd., London

Library of Congress Cataloging-in-Publication Data
McIntyre, Anne.
the medicinal garden: how to grow and use your own medicinal herbs –
Anne McIntyre.
p.   cm.
"An Owl book."
Includes index.
1. Materia medica, Vegetable.   2. Herbs—Therapeutic use.
I. Title
RS 164. M352   1997   96-41112
615'.321—dc 20   CIP

ISBN 0-8050-4838-3

First American Edition—1997

Designed by Roger Daniels

Printed in Hong Kong
All first editions are printed on acid-free paper.
1   3   5   7   9   10   8   6   4   2   ∞

CONTENTS

Introduction
～ 6 ～

GROWING MEDICINAL PLANTS
～ 13 ～

PREPARING HERBAL REMEDIES
～ 33 ～

A-Z OF MEDICINAL PLANTS:
The Cultivated Garden
～ 43 ～

A-Z OF MEDICINAL PLANTS:
The Wild Garden
～ 112 ～

HERB & AILMENT CHART
～ 126 ～

Glossary
～ 148 ～

Seed Companies & Nurseries
～ 149 ～

Index
～ 150 ～

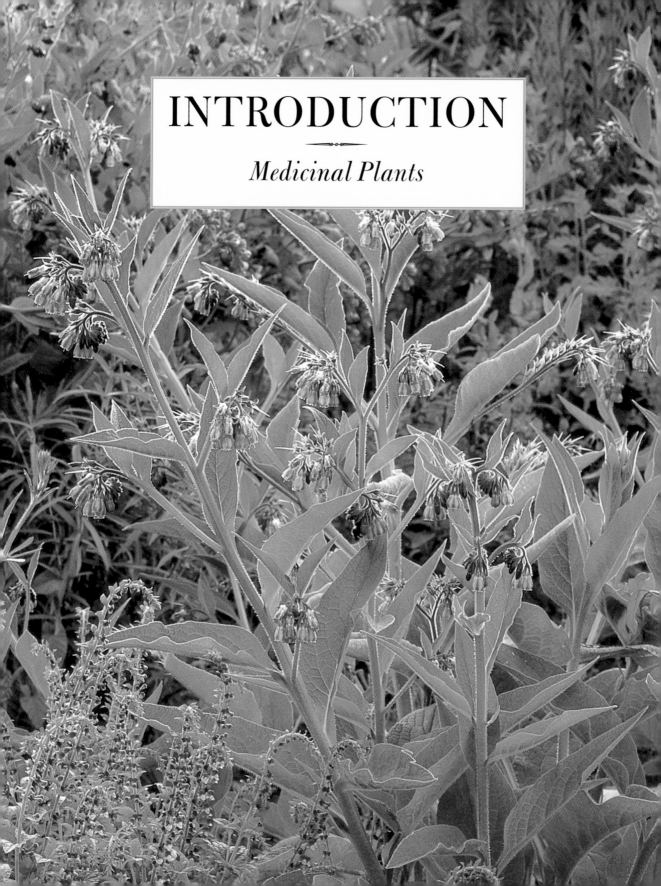

INTRODUCTION

Medicinal Plants

Though a life of retreat offers various joys,
None, I think, will compare with the time one
employs,
In the study of herbs, or in striving to gain
Some practical knowledge of Nature's
Domain.
Get a garden!

HORTULUS OR THE LITTLE GARDEN,
WALAFRID STRABO AD 900

The garden is a healing place. If you have a love of plants and gardening then you will know the sense of joy and serenity that can be derived from a few hours spent in the garden, tending your plants or simply relaxing and reflecting on the beauty around you. For many the garden is their sanctuary, a place of peace and refreshment away from the rush and stress of everyday life. It can be a haven for recreation and meditation, offering a sense of closeness to Nature.

The first gardens of western civilisation were created when people started to settle in communities and needed to grow plants to provide food and medicines. The oldest pictures of gardens that exist are from ancient Egypt, dating around 1400 BC. Such gardens were surrounded by walls or palisades to protect them from desert winds and thieves. Fruit trees and plants, both nutritious and medicinal, were laid out in symmetrical shapes and rows interspersed with waterways to ease irrigation. Despite being predominantly utilitarian, they were also highly decorative.

Early gardens represented the contrast between two different worlds. Outside the garden untamed nature was all-powerful and potentially threatening, while, inside the enclosure, not only was safety offered but trees provided cool shade, and water

sustained the plants and restored the soul. As time went by, the enclosed garden came to symbolise the joys of paradise. The early gardens of the Islamic world were highly sophisticated, and the ancient Persian name for such gardens was *pairidaeza*, from which we get the word 'paradise'. It was taken into Old Testament Hebrew as *pardes* and into Greek as *paradeisos*, by which time it meant a royal and beautiful garden or park. In later Hebrew it represented both the Garden of Eden, the source of all creation, and the kingdom of heaven or celestial paradise, the home of the angels and saints and the abode of the virtuous after death.

To the early Christians the enclosed garden – *hortulus conclusus* – symbolised the feminine in nature, the purity of a virgin and the womb for the conception and growth of everything that lives. The garden was the purity of the virgin bride of Solomon's *Song of Songs*:

A garden enclosed is my sister, my spouse,
A spring shut up, a fountain sealed.

The Virgin Mary was described as the 'fountain of gardens' and Dante called her a 'fountain of living things' to wash away the sins of the world and confer grace. In medieval days, Mary gardens were decorated with flowers dedicated to the Virgin Mary, such as lady's mantle, lavender, rosemary, chamomile, daisies, violets and marigolds.

The Christian Church applied the old enclosed garden design of the Middle East to the round or semi-circular garden by the walls of the monastery or cathedral. This was actually known as 'the paradise' and usually tended by the sacrist who grew plants there which had religious significance for decorating the church on special occasions. The cloister garden was larger, planted with aromatic herbs which scented the air and enhanced the tranquillity of the monk's place of study and meditation as well as serving more practical purposes.

The world of plants not only offered a glimpse of the realms of paradise, but it also provided for a wide range of earthly needs. Since the beginning of time people have depended on plants for food, clothing, shelter, fodder and fuel. Certain plants also offered protection against the known and the unkown – the powers of darkness and the evil eye which threatened our ancestors. Plants provide the oxygen we breathe and for thousands of years have given us medicines for almost every ill. Remedies derived from plants have been used for healing both the body and the soul.

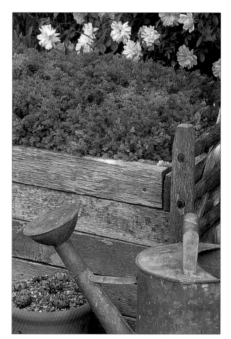

We can trace the connection between human existence and healing herbs to Neanderthal man. In 1963 in Iraq archeologists opened the grave of a man in a cave who had been buried 60,000 years ago with several herbs, most probably for their symbolic and healing significance. We know that as far back as 3000 BC schools of herbal medicine existed in Egypt, China, Assyria and India. The earliest written records of herbal medicine are the Chinese treatises attributed to the Yellow Emperor around 2,500 BC called the *Pen T'Sao*, and the Ebers papyrus of 1,500 BC which describes symptoms and their treatments using over 700 herbs including mint, senna, gentian, poppy, dill, lettuce and the castor oil plant.

Hippocrates (468-377 BC), the first important medical thinker of the West, recorded his 'humoral theory' and the use of over 400 medicinal plants. His work was later developed by Artistotle and Theophrastus. Their writings, together with the celebrated herbal of Dioscorides, *De Materia Medica*, written in the 2nd century AD and describing over 500 plants, became the foundation of European medicine. From about the 4th century onwards, knowledge of medicinal plants was kept alive predominantly within the medieval monasteries, which were the main storehouses of knowledge. Monks copied and recopied texts of the classic herbals from ancient Greek and Latin and illustrated them with woodcuts, often bearing little resemblance to the original plants.

Most monasteries had to be self-sufficient, growing food in one area of the garden and medicinal plants to supply the infirmary in another. The oldest preserved plan of an ideal monastery garden, probably designed by Abbot Reichenau in the 9th century, was discovered at the Benedictine monastery of St Gall in Switzerland. The physic garden was situated by the physician's house and the infirmary, and was divided into sixteen parallel beds planted with healing herbs including fennel, mint, rose, rosemary, sage and savory. Although this plan may never have been actually created its style clearly influenced garden design throughout the next few centuries. Herbs grown especially for their healing benefits in such gardens gained the suffix *officinale*.

Other herbal knowledge was passed down by oral tradition from one generation to another. It was usually women who were the herb gatherers, and neighbouring families relied heavily on the skills of such 'wise women' particularly if the nearest monastery was some distance away. The

oldest surviving English herbal, now in the British Library, *The Leech Book of Bald,* dates from Anglo-Saxon times. It was compiled by a scribe called Cild under the direction of a monk called Bald, who was a contemporary of King Alfred. It gives prescriptions and describes the herbal lore of familiar herbs such as vervain, wood betony, periwinkles and violets.

The invention of the printing press in the 15th century revolutionised the spread of herbal information in Europe. Old hand-copied herbals were replaced by printed books which were more widely available to medical students and those studying plants. The new spirit of learning of the Renaissance encouraged direct observation and drawing of plants from nature. The

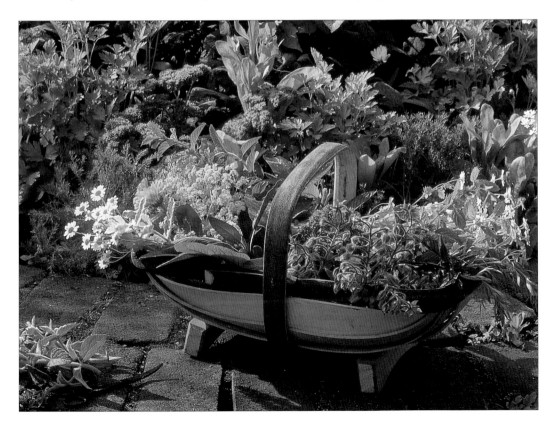

science of botany began to develop as a study of the plants themselves rather than of their medicinal properties.

A great number of new herbals began to appear around this time, notably those of Gerard and Culpeper, still popular today. In 1596 John Gerard, herbalist to James I, catalogued 1030 plants in his London garden; he published his *Herball* in 1597. Culpeper's *English Physician*, published in 1652, related herbs and the symptoms of the body to stars and planets. John Parkinson's herbals, *Paradisi in Sole Paradisus Terrestris* (1629) – a pun on his name 'Park in Sun's Earthly Paradise' – and *Theatrum Botanicum* (1640) were among the last publications to combine all aspects of plant knowledge – botany, pharmacy, horticulture and history – under one title.

At this time plants needed by physicians for medicinal purposes and for the teaching of their students were grown together in physic gardens. The first such comprehensive collections of medicinal plants were established in Italy, first in Pisa (1543), then in Padua (1545) and Florence (1550). Other countries soon followed suit, in Leipzig (1580), Heidelberg (1593) and Paris (1635). In Britain the first university medicinal herb garden was founded in 1621 in Oxford for the study of herbs, while Edinburgh's physic garden was planted in 1656 for the teaching of surgeons and apothecaries. Doctors were appointed to lecture at universities on the healing properties of herbs. Chelsea Physic Garden was established in 1673 for apprentices of the Society of Apothecaries for the 'manifestation of the glory, power and wisdom of God, in the works of creation'. Until the Embankment was built in the 1870s, the garden ran right down to the Thames and the apprentices were frequently brought by barge during their nine years' training. John Evelyn, the 17th-century diarist, called the Chelsea Physic Garden 'the Apothecaries' Garden of Simples'. Nearly all the existing botanic gardens started as physic gardens.

In the late 16th and early 17th centuries, gardens became inundated with new exotic species brought almost daily by navigators and explorers from abroad, and at the same time attitudes towards plants and gardens began to change considerably. The new spirit of scientific analysis attacked traditional rituals associated with the prescribing of herbs, as they smacked of mysticism, even sorcery, rather than the workings of the rational scientific mind. Doctors began to rely on other, often toxic, substances such as mercury and arsenic, as well as blood-letting, for their treatments.

Until this time, herbs had not been grown separately from ornamental plants, for almost all cultivated plants possessed culinary or medicinal virtues, or were used in a symbolic way, such as for protection against evil, or conferring the spiritual protection of the Virgin Mary. Even their beauty had healing effects, enhancing general health and well-being by awakening the spirit and enriching the soul. By the 18th century medicinal herbs were generally grown away from the purely decorative plants in the ornamental garden, reflecting the philosophy of the day, of the separation of man and nature, mind and body. In the contemporary mechanistic theory, nature was no longer perceived as alive and inextricably linked with human life on all levels, but as an inanimate source of natural resources, to be plundered for economic development. Herbs were mostly banished to the kitchen garden, although they did remain in the traditional cottage gardens in medleys of fruit, flowers, vegetables and herbs, to be used by the 'old wives' for the everyday ills of country folk.

As herbalism was going into decline in Europe it was being developed in America. The seeds and roots of medicinal herbs and copies of the great herbals of the day accompanied the first colonists to America. Their ships returned with Native American wisdom and plants to be grown and studied in European physic gardens. The early settlers adopted Native American remedies from herbs such as echinacea, black cohosh and witch hazel, which are still favourites among herbalists today.

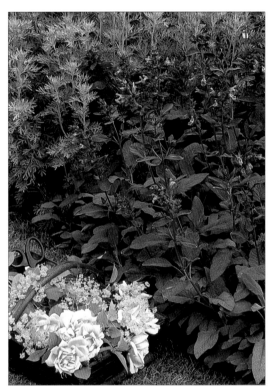

The first American botanic garden was founded near Philadelphia in 1728, by John Bartram, a botanist who regularly sent plants back to London. Over the next century, lack of confidence in orthodox physicians using toxic substances and blood-letting gave rise to a demand for herbal patent medicines and a flourishing herb industry began to develop. The Shakers, a religious group who used diet, faith and herbal medicine to keep their members well, were among those to establish a successful herbal business, and in 1820 they created the first of many medicinal herb gardens in New York.

At the end of the 19th century, however, the demand for herbal medicines in Western Europe diminished still further, thanks to the rapid developments of the Industrial Revolution and discoveries in the world of science. Nature was seen simply in terms of its exploitation to enable technological and economic progress and as a source of chemical constituents. Herbalism was fast becoming obsolete and in gardens all but the culinary elite of herbs – parsley, rosemary, sage, thyme, marjoram and bay – together with a few favourite ornamental herbs, such as lavender, rapidly became unfashionable.

It was not until the 1960s that positive change was in the air with the emergence of environmental consciousness and 'flower power'. Increasing recognition that good diet and lifestyle are the basis for health, along with the growing disenchantment with fast foods, artificial additives and the overuse of powerful drugs for minor ills, has reinstated the role of herbs in diet and general health. An interesting variety of culinary herbs enhances our increasingly cosmopolitan and adventurous cuisine, while in many homes herbs are being used to treat common ailments and in most pharmacies a range of herbal medicines is likely to be found.

Today, both philosophers and scientists are adopting a more holistic approach to the study of the relationship between self and body, human beings and nature. The earth and all plant, animal and human life on it are again being perceived as one vast living organism, a self-organising and self-regulating system. This ancient idea, clearly propounded by the British scientist James Lovelock in the 1970s as the Gaia hypothesis, reflects the medieval concepts of microcosm and macrocosm, the astrological approach to herbs and the body set out by Culpeper and many before him including Hippocrates, and the humoral philosophy of Hippocrates and his followers.

Such philosophical shifts are being reflected in the garden. Herbs are being reinstated from their lowly position in the corner of the vegetable patch to enhance flower borders and even warrant whole gardens of their own. Many gardeners now buy plants not only for their decorative attributes but for their magical, romantic, symbolic, medicinal and historical associations. Growing such herbs is an excellent way to acquaint yourself more fully with plants that are not only beautiful and aromatic but also effective medicines. Your garden can be your instant medicine cabinet, enabling you to treat a wide range of everyday minor ailments such as coughs and colds, catarrh, stomach aches, headaches, and other aches and pains, thereby reducing visits to your doctor and curbing the use of powerful medicines for minor self-limiting illness. Tending your herb garden may

stimulate your curiosity and lead you to discover how many common garden plants or even nuisance 'weeds' are valuable herbal remedies and have potent therapeutic compounds. Pasque flowers, pansies, roses, dandelions and even couch grass spring instantly to mind. Apparently simple herbs that grow easily in most soils have warranted much time and money invested in current research as to their potential use in curing illness such as viral infection, immune deficiency, malaria, peptic ulcers and many acute and degenerative as well as stress-related disorders; such herbs include echinacea, St John's wort, artemisia annua and liquorice. A medicinal garden can contain those healing plants from all over the world that will grow in a temperate climate such as those used in Chinese medicine – bamboo, peony, wisteria and balloon flowers – or those found in Native American medicine – Joe Pye weed, skullcap and black cohosh.

By creating a medicinal or apothecary's garden you will be following in the footsteps of many an eminent herbalist and herb gardener of the past. Plants that have been grown by priests, physicians and apothecaries through millennia are little changed today – cowslips, violets and roses, for example, are as popular in herb gardens today as they were a thousand years ago in monastery gardens. Such plants and gardens connect us through centuries of existence to men and women who have gardened, cooked and healed with these plants and gazed on them with wonder and delight as we do now. They represent a living history, connecting us to a time when plants were valued not only for their earthly gifts but also for their spiritual benefits. They can still provide a glimpse of paradise.

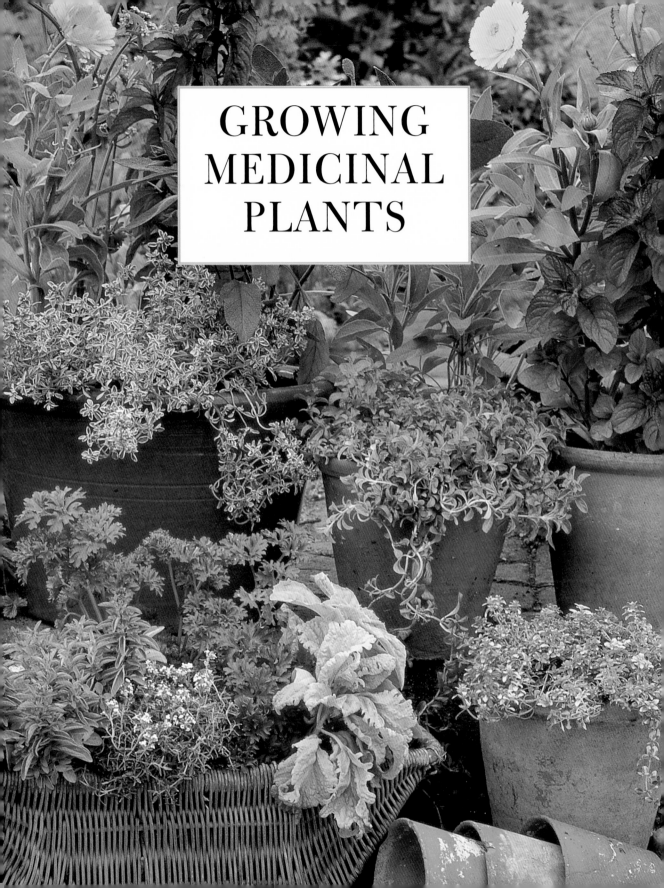

GROWING MEDICINAL PLANTS

Herbs are wonderfully rewarding plants to grow. Providing they have suitable soil and shelter from prevailing winds, most medicinal herbs are easy to grow, with no specialist knowledge or skills required. A herb garden can be as large or small, as formal or informal as you wish. Herbs can be planted in specially designed herb gardens, in herbaceous borders, in corners of vegetable gardens, or intermingled with the vegetables, in pots on a patio and also in window boxes or pots on your windowsill. Both the planning and the practical laying out of a herb garden can bring many hours of pleasure and satisfaction.

Planning your herb garden

Many of the herbs we know and those used as medicines originate in warm climates, so in order to grow happily in cool temperate

HERB BORDER

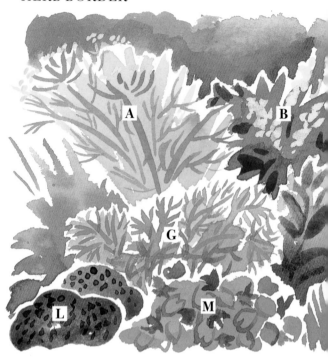

SOIL

When planning your garden, you will need to make sure that the type of soil is suitable for the herbs you intend to plant. It there is adequate top soil with reasonable drainage, those plants which thrive in moist loamy soils will grow well in clay.

Moist loam	Well-drained loam	Chalky soil	Light sandy soil	Clay soil	Marshy ground
angelica	bay	catmint/catnip	chamomile	burdock	angelica
chives	basil	hyssop	coriander/	comfrey	comfrey
comfrey	burdock	lavender	cilantro	mints	mints
elecampane	catmint/catnip	lungwort	fennel	wormwood	marsh mallow
lady's mantle	coriander/	marjoram	lavender		meadowsweet
lemon balm	cilantro	motherwort	thyme		skullcap
lovage	dill	pasque flower	wild carrot		valerian
meadowsweet	fennel	rosemary			
mints	hyssop				
parsley	juniper				
skullcap	lady's mantle				
soapwort	lavender				
sweet violet	lovage				
valerian	marjoram				
	rosemary				
	rue				
	sage				
	thyme				

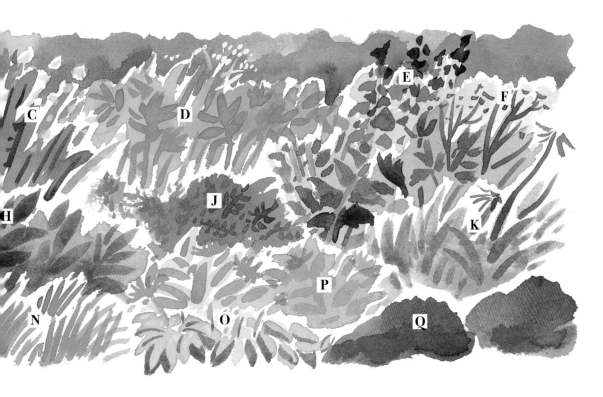

climes they prefer a sheltered position. If your garden is warm and sheltered there is no need to be concerned about enclosing it and herbs can be planted in the open. Otherwise, a hedge or fence suitably sited for their protection will have the added advantage of allowing the fragrances of the herbs to linger on warm air, rather than being blown away from a breezy open position.

Before planting your herb garden it is a good idea to sit down with a pen and paper and make rough plans of your garden and planting design. First of all you need to decide where you will allocate your herb garden, or decide on the space where you will grow your herbs. Siting herbs near the house has its advantages, as it is easy to harvest them, and harder to forget what you

Key to Plants

A	Fennel	**J**	Black cohosh
B	Meadowsweet	**K**	Echinacea
C	Mullein	**L**	Thyme
D	Angelica	**M**	Violets
E	Hollyhock	**N**	Chives
F	Lovage	**O**	Cowslip
G	Wormwood	**P**	Marigold
H	Purple sage	**Q**	Heather

have and let the herbs go over before you notice them. You will also see and appreciate their appearance and delicious scents the nearer you have them to the house. You also need to take into account your type of soil (*see page* 14), and the aspect of the site, related to the amount of sun or shade. Although herbs like to be grown in warm, sheltered and sunny positions, some prefer light shade, so your herb-growing area should ideally include a shady area – often provided by a hedge or fence.

Herbs in herbaceous borders

A walled garden is an ideal place for a herb border – or a herbaceous border with a mixture of herbs, shrubs and flowers. Without a wall, you may need a hedge or fence to provide shelter for your border.

Hedging behind the border should be evergreen and dark-leaved, not only to provide shelter but also to provide a dense, dark background to show off the fine and lighter coloured and silvery herbs to best advantage. When choosing hedging plants, it is important not to choose shrubs or small trees that take too much moisture or nutrients from the soil, such as privet. Ideal plants are those that can be controlled easily by clipping such as bay, myrtle and juniper. Young bay and myrtle may need some protection during a cold winter and are best grown on a sheltered site with their roots protected. In a small border dwarf juniper (*J. communis* 'compressa') would work well

as it grows in a narrow column, takes up little space and creates minimal shade.

Fencing at the back of the border may be your preferred option. It enables climbing plants (such as jasmine, roses, honeysuckle and hops) to be displayed to advantage. Fencing is relatively cheap to erect and provides instant shelter which could make all the difference in an open and exposed garden as to whether your herbs survive and flourish. Remember that either a fence or a hedge will give some shade to the border which will mean that you will be able to plant both shade- and sun-loving plants.

Choose the herbs that you like best for your herb border, and make a list of them. When deciding on their positions in the border, check their height and the time of year when they will look interesting and decorative, to ensure interest in your border for as long as possible through the changing seasons.

Low-growing plants such as marjoram, violets, thyme, chives, marigolds, pennyroyal, pasque flower, heather and cowslip will obviously be best planted near

---

CHOOSING PLANTS

Size, shape and texture are important considerations when choosing plants for a herbaceous border. Small, delicate plants with fine, feathery foliage make an excellent contrast with tall, large-leaved plants.

Bold architectural plants	Soft-coloured, delicate or fluffy foliage	Fine-leaved, or feathery plants	Tall, large-leaved plants
angelica	catmint/catnip	chamomile	angelica
burdock	lady's mantle	coriander/cilantro	burdock
clary sage	marjoram	dill	clary sage
comfrey	marsh mallow	fennel	comfrey
elecampane	rue	hyssop	globe artichoke
fennel	soapwort	lavender	horseradish
globe artichoke	valerian	parsley	lovage
horseradish	wormwood	rue	mullein
lovage		southernwood	marsh mallow
meadowsweet		valerian	
milk thistle		wormwood	
		yarrow	

LADDER DESIGN HERB BORDER

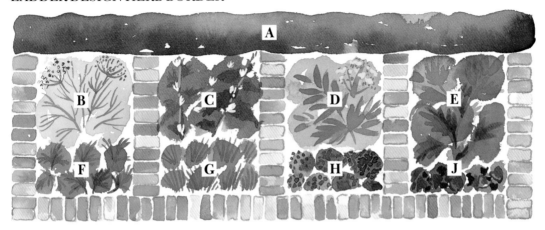

the front, and taller ones such as lovage, angelica, borage, comfrey, elecampane and fennel should go at the back. If the border is large, herbs are best planted in clumps or drifts as Gertrude Jekyll preferred, rather than singly, for greater visual effect. If you choose herbs that quickly grow into good clumps, you will find that relatively soon after planting, even within a few summer months, your garden will start to look quite full and established. Herbs such as sage,

Key to Plants

A	Hedge – myrtle or juniper	**E**	Lovage
B	Fennel	**F**	Parsley
C	Marshmallow	**G**	Chives
D	Angelica	**H**	Thyme
		J	Violets

betony, thyme, rosemary and hyssop establish themselves surprisingly quickly. Some herbs are best planted in groups of three to five in order to give a good show – for example, greater celandine, clary sage, meadowsweet, gentian, echinacea, black cohosh, bistort, marigolds, violets and nasturtiums. Others that are shrubby or large and expansive are better planted singly; these include mullein, rosemary, sage, southernwood, wormwood, lavender, lovage, angelica and fennel. While there are gaps between perennials in the first year or two, annual herbs such as dill, marigolds and basil can be planted.

To give your border a more formal feel, you could edge it with low-growing herbs such as thyme, golden marjoram, pennyroyal or chamomile, or a low-growing hedge of dwarf lavender, hyssop, rosemary or

POSITION

The aspect of the site should be taken into account when choosing plants for your garden. Although most herbs like to grow in warm, sheltered and sunny positions, some prefer light shade, so your herb garden should include a shady patch – often provided by the proximity of a hedge or fence.

Full sun	Dappled shade	Shade
basil	angelica	comfrey
bay	chives	lungwort
coriander/	fennel	mint
cilantro	ground ivy	valerian
hyssop	lemon balm	violet
lavender	lovage	
marjoram	mint	
rosemary	parsley	
sage	wild	
thyme	strawberry	

southernwood. Alternatively you can design your border as a more informal, cottage-type garden, and create a wonderfully exuberant confusion of shape, colour and aroma. Such a garden can occur with little planning, almost by instinct or good luck, or it can be the result of over-planting, where a profusion of herbs jostle for space and light. But if it doesn't work it can look messy, so it may well be a better idea to work out your plant positions and happy combinations and companions before planting.

Once your herbs are established and growing well, the border should give little trouble and require a minimum of maintenance during the growing season. So that it does not look empty and too bleak in winter, it is a good idea to intersperse herbaceous herbs with evergreen shrubs, or shrubs with winter interest such as bright red berries of cramp bark, purple berries of juniper bushes, or with winter flowering shrubs such as witch hazel.

FORMAL HERB GARDEN DESIGNS

When planning and designing a more formal or traditional herb garden, it is important to keep the pattern simple for best effect. The shape should be regular and symmetrical – round, square or rectangular – divided into a number of distinguishable, equal sections to form a repetitive pattern, with a focal point in the centre, such as a sundial, fountain or pool, a statue or statuesque plant such as angelica, or a small area of chamomile lawn.

First of all measure the plot for your herb garden and then plan it on paper before marking it out with powdered chalk or flour on the ground. Map out its shape and paths or divisions between sections. Make sure

KNOT GARDEN: INTERLEAVED SHAMROCK DESIGN

Key to Plants
A Marigolds
B Rosemary
C Sage
D Lemon balm
E Marjoram
F Hyssop
G Chives
H Thyme
J Dwarf nasturtiums
K Parlsey

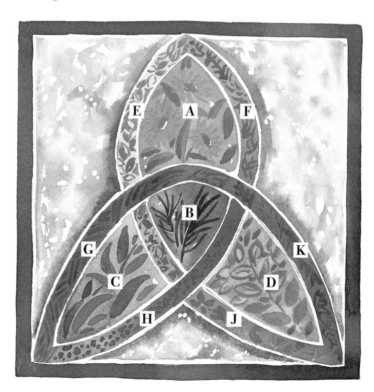

KNOT GARDEN: LOZENGE DESIGN

Key to Plants
A Wormwood
B Hyssop
C Box hedge
D Lavender
E Gravel

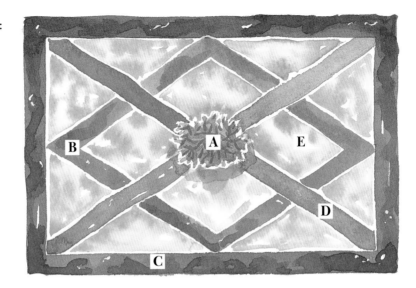

what type of soil the area has and how much sunlight/shade it has before selecting plants for it. The basis of your design will be the paths – grass, gravel, brick or paved – which are vital for providing access to each herb bed. When planting keep it simple.

In a formal garden, edging plants or low hedges lining the paths give a good effect. Herbs that can be easily clipped to keep their shape such as lavender, hyssop or rosemary are best for a formal hedge. Buy young evenly shaped plants and plant them in well-dug fertile soil, with plenty of manure or garden compost for extra nourishment. After planting, prune back to encourage bushy new growth at the base of each plant. As the plants develop, trim back side-shoots to keep the hedge compact and cut the tops to give the hedge a neat finish.

The Knot Garden

You may like to incorporate formal designs from the past into your herb garden plan. Monastic herb gardens of the Middle Ages were enclosed by formal hedges and geometrically criss-crossed with paths to make the herbs easily available to the herb gatherers. In Tudor and Elizabethan times, the heyday of the apothecaries, knot gardens became highly popular. Low-growing hedging plants such as box, hyssop and lavender were grown in interwoven lines, resembling the pattern made by a knotted rope. Though such complicated designs are very attractive, their maintenance requires the devotion of a very dedicated gardener with plenty of time on his or her hands! However, a more simple modern knot garden could be designed along traditional lines, as shown here.

The Physic Garden

The 16th century apothecary or 'physic' gardens were frequently planted close to an infirmary, where apothecaries mixed their tinctures and ointments. Physic gardens later became established as collections of scientifically and medically valued herbs known as botanic gardens. They were often laid out very formally in rectangular beds, in which plants were arranged in methodical order and regular patterns.

THEMATIC PLANT GROUPING: BODY SYSTEMS

When planting your medicinal garden you will find you are spoilt for choice, for among medicinal herbs are some of the most beautiful and interesting in the plant world.

Thematic groupings, according to the system of the body the herbs benefit, might be one way of arranging such a garden.

Respiratory system	Digestive system	Urinary system	Nervous system	Reproductive system	Skin
coneflower	angelica	burdock	catmint/catnip	blessed thistle	burdock
elder	chamomile	chamomile	chamomile	chamomile	chickweed
elecampane	coriander/	fennel	cowslip	clary sage	comfrey
garlic	cilantro	heather	dill	hops	dandelion
ground ivy	dill	Joe Pye weed	hops	lady's mantle	dock
horehound	fennel	marsh mallow	jasmine	marigold	elderflower
hyssop	garlic	meadowsweet	lemon balm	motherwort	figwort
mullein	hops	nettle	pasque flower	pasque flower	fumitory
lavender	lemon balm	parsley	rose	periwinkle	lavender
lungwort	lovage	plantain	rosemary	rose	liquorice
rose	marsh mallow	vervain	skullcap	sage	marigold
sage	meadowsweet	wild carrot	valerian	southernwood	marsh mallow
thyme	mint		vervain	thyme	nettle
	rosemary		wild oats	wormwood	plantain
	sage		wood betony		rose
	thyme				wild pansy
	vervain				
	wormwood				
	yarrow				

THEMATIC PLANT GROUPING: HEALING PROPERTIES

You will find that the same herb will crop up when considering different body systems. Choose where you feel the herb looks best in relation to other herbs you have chosen, and put it in one section only to avoid confusion. You could also group herbs according to their healing properties:

Astringent	Demulcent (soothing)	Anti-spasmodic	Diuretic	Antiseptic	Circulatory stimulant	Relaxant	Alterative	First-aid
agrimony	clary sage	angelica	burdock	basil	angelica	basil	burdock	agrimony
bistort	comfrey	basil	chamomile	bay	garlic	chamomile	cleavers	burdock
lady's	flax	catmint/	cleavers	chamomile	hawthorn	clary sage	dandelion	comfrey
mantle	liquorice	catnip	dandelion	coneflower	horseradish	cowslip	elderflower	dock
marigold	lungwort	chamomile	fennel	fennel	juniper	hops	figwort	garlic
periwinkle	marsh	coriander/	heather	garlic	peppermint	jasmine	fumitory	lavender
rose	mallow	cilantro	Joe Pye	hyssop	rosemary	lemon balm	marigold	marigold
tormentil	mullein	dill	weed	juniper	thyme	pasque	nettles	plantain
wildstraw-	plantain	elecampane	lovage	lavender	yarrow	flower	plantain	St John's
berry		fennel	meadow-	lemon balm		rose	rose	wort
witch hazel		hyssop	sweet	marigold		skullcap	vervain	witch hazel
yarrow		lavender	nettles	marjoram		St John's	wild pansy	yarrow
		lemon balm	parsley	mint		wort	wormwood	
		lovage	plantain	parsley		valerian		
		mint	vervain	rose		vervain		
		rosemary		rosemary		wild oats		
		yarrow		sage		wood		
				thyme		betony		

PHYSIC GARDEN – MEDICINE WHEELS

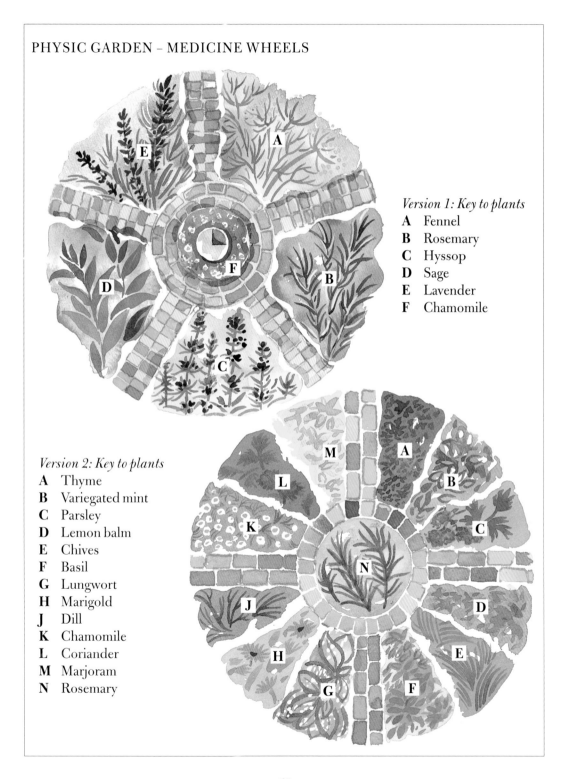

Version 1: Key to plants
A   Fennel
B   Rosemary
C   Hyssop
D   Sage
E   Lavender
F   Chamomile

Version 2: Key to plants
A   Thyme
B   Variegated mint
C   Parsley
D   Lemon balm
E   Chives
F   Basil
G   Lungwort
H   Marigold
J   Dill
K   Chamomile
L   Coriander
M   Marjoram
N   Rosemary

Many modern herb garden designs can look just as effective as the knot or physic gardens. A good place to start is with a circle divided into wedge shapes around a central focus, like a wheel (*see page* 21). This can look attractive and is relatively simple to design and create. If you have plenty of space and want to create a more intricate design with a greater variety of herbs, some of the more complex and ambitious designs may be of interest.

The medicinal garden could be aptly enclosed by a hedge of the apothecary's rose, *Rosa gallica*, or with shrubby hedges of rosemary, hyssop or lavender.

The Aromatic Garden
It is hard to imagine anything more delightful than walking among a melody of scents, brushing against aromatic leaves of coriander, lemon balm, mint, rosemary, sage or wormwood, walking on a scented thyme, chamomile or mint lawn, or inhaling the heady scent of roses, honeysuckle, jasmine, lavender or evening primrose. Smells are evocative and stirring, and have been used for thousands of years to heal us on mental and emotional as well as physiological levels. Flowers and leaves have been the source of scents to adorn the body, to enhance religious ceremonies and to protect against evil, each aroma having a different specific action. It is important to choose herbs whose scent you love (*see page 24*).

The aroma of scented plants is derived from volatile oils present in flowers and leaves. The tiny oil-secreting glands can often be seen as tiny pin-prick dots when the leaf is held up to the light. The oils are released when the flowers or leaves are brushed against or bruised. This needs to be borne in mind when planting aromatic herbs

PHYSIC GARDEN – FORMAL LAYOUT

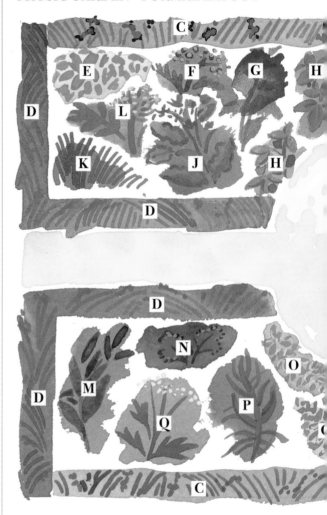

as they have to be near or overhanging paths for people to come into contact with them. Some scents, such as those of chamomile, lemon balm and rosemary, are released only if the plant is crushed, as the oil-containing glands are contained deep within the plant's structure, while others, such as angelica, elderflower, lavender and thyme, are more superficial and their aromas are released just by the warmth of the sun. An aromatic

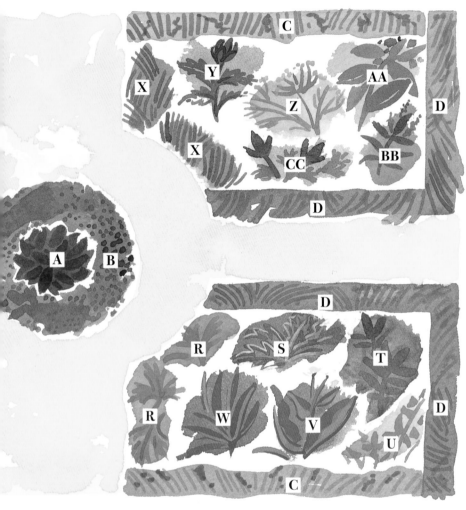

Key to Plants:
A   Bay tree
B   Creeping
    thyme
C   Hyssop
D   Lavender
E   Apple Mint
F   Lovage
G   Skullcap
H   Wild
    Strawberry
J   Borage
K   Lemon balm
L   Angelica
M   Sage
N   Coriander
O   Sweet
    Marjoram
P   Tarragon
Q   Lovage
R   Parsley
S   Milk thistle
T   Meadowsweet
U   St John's wort
V   Elecampane
W   Echinacea
X   Chives
Y   Globe
    artichoke
Z   Fennel
AA Variegated
    comfrey
BB Black cohosh
CC Pasque flower

garden needs to be interspersed with several paths at short intervals to allow close proximity with scented plants. A seat or arbor nearby with trailing or climbing aromatic plants such as roses, honeysuckle, jasmine and hops would be ideal. The aromatic garden needs to be sited in a particularly sheltered area to enable scents to linger in the air.

Among the paving stones in paths, or used instead of grass lawn in paths, patios and around garden seats, creeping aromatic plants such as chamomile, pennyroyal, wild thyme or yarrow can be delightful, as they release their aroma everytime someone steps on them.

Hedges around the beds or the circumference of the garden can add not only to the structure and design of the garden but also to its mixture of fragrances, releasing their aroma when anyone brushes past them. Choose from hyssop, lavender, rose, rosemary or southernwood.

The Wild Herb Garden

If you have room, the creation of a wild herb garden will offer sanctuary to many of the wild herbs currently under threat from chemical sprays, pollution and the destruction of their natural habitat. An area under a deciduous tree, such as a cherry or apple tree, is a good area for a patch of wild garden. In a larger area of meadow, paths mown among tall grass and meadow flowers enable you to appreciate their colours and scent and to check that they are not getting lost or smothered.

To plant a wild garden

Wild herb seed and meadow flower seed can be bought and grown in seed trays. Once the plants are ready to plant out in grassland, lift a large piece of turf for each one, dig a hole larger than is needed and fill it with plenty of good, fine-textured loam. Water the plants and keep an eye on them until they are well established. Check that the ground does not dry out in hot weather and that neighbouring grasses do not completely smother the new plants. By autumn of the same year

resilient perennials such as agrimony, dock, plantain, nettles, cleavers, comfrey, dandelion and horseradish should be able to cope with competition. Biennials such as mullein, wild carrot and burdock should self-seed, but it is worth collecting some seed just in case. Less aggressive plants such as violets, cowslips, wild strawberry and wood betony may need more attention.

Another way of planting a wild area is to buy wild herb seed already mixed with grass seed, or to mix it yourself. Clear the ground

---

PLANTS THAT CAN GROW WILD

agrimony	ground ivy	plantain
bistort	hawthorn	St John's wort
burdock	honeysuckle	tormentil
chickweed	hops	violets
cleavers	horseradish	wild carrot
comfrey	lungwort	wild pansy
cowslips	marjoram	wild
dandelion	marsh mallow	strawberry
dock	meadowsweet	wood betony
elderflowers	mullein	yarrow
figwort	nettle	
fumitory	pasque flower	

HERBS FOR AROMATHERAPY

Herb	Aromatic Property
angelica	warming, uplifting, strengthening, invigorating
basil	uplifting, calming, pain-relieving, antiseptic
chamomile	calming, sleep inducing, pacifying, pain-relieving
clary sage	relaxing, uplifting even euphoric
coriander/cilantro	invigorating, stimulating, pain-relieving
fennel	cleansing, refreshing, relaxing
honeysuckle	calming, relaxing, romantic
hops	calming, sleep-inducing, relaxing and mentally strengthening
jasmine	calming, uplifting, reassuring, sensual
lavender	calming and balancing, pain-relieving, insect repellent
lemon balm	calming and uplifting and strengthening, insect repellent
marjoram	strengthening, calming, comforting
mint	clears the head, pain-relieving, refreshing, awakening
rose	relaxing, calming, comforting, sensual, uplifting, cleansing
rosemary	uplifting, invigorating and strengthening
southernwood	increases awareness
thyme	invigorating, strengthening, antiseptic, insect repellent, warming
violet	uplifting, sleep-inducing, calming, soothing and cooling

AROMATIC GARDEN

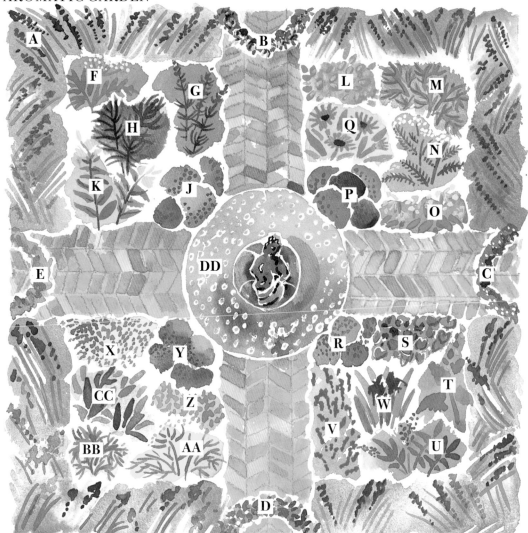

Key to Plants:

A	Lavender hedge	**K**	Evening primrose	**U**	Meadowsweet
B	Climbing honeysuckle	**L**	Lemon balm	**V**	Catmint
C	Climbing Jasmine	**M**	Wormwood	**W**	Iris
D	Climbing roses	**N**	Yarrow	**X**	Pennyroyal
E	Climbing hops	**O**	Cowslip	**Y**	Thyme
F	Angelica	**P**	Thyme	**Z**	Oregano
G	Hyssop	**Q**	Marigold	**AA**	Fennel
H	Rosemary	**R**	Thyme	**BB**	Southernwood
J	Thyme	**S**	Violets	**CC**	Sage
		T	Clary sage	**DD**	Chamomile

of weeds, dig it well, level it and sow seed as you would for a lawn. Keep the area watered well in dry weather until growth is well established. The toughest will survive while some of the less forceful herbs may get lost.

A wild garden can look very attractive by early to midsummer. Once all the flowers have gone over and seeds have dropped, the garden can be scythed down to about 20cm (8in) high.

HERBS IN THE VEGETABLE GARDEN

Herbs look very decorative planted in a corner here and there in the vegetable garden, or in rows interspersed among the vegetables. Using herbs as edging can give a vegetable garden the appearance of a parterre garden – parsley, lavender, chives, dill, southernwood, marigolds, thyme, or hyssop will make either neat rows or low growing hedges for edging.

Companion planting

Aromatic herbs in the vegetable garden have long been known for their beneficial effects on the growth and health of their companion vegetables, all except fennel, which can retard the growth of beans, tomatoes and kohlrabi. Stinging nettles growing near aromatic herbs increase the strength of their aroma by increasing their essential oil content. Yarrow acts similarly.

Some herbs high in essential oils give off such strong aromas that they disguise the smell of neighbouring plants and thus protect them from predators. Others secrete substances from their roots into the soil that benefit their neighbours, or have such deep roots that they bring nutrients up to the more superficial soil and they help break up heavy soil. Chamomile and borage increase resistance to disease. Coriander hinders the

seed formation of fennel but attracts bees to the garden when it is in bloom, and fennel does not grow well near wormwood. Tall resilient plants protect smaller/more delicate ones from wind, sun and cold. Some are very popular with moths, bees and other insects, bringing pollinators to the area. All herbs grow more quickly and healthily together, rather than when planted singly, so the more variation in plants grown together the better.

Insect-repellent herbs

Certain herbs make excellent companion plants because they have the ability to repel insects when several are planted in the vicinity. Basil around a rose bush, for example, will keep aphids away and feverfew around a bed of carrots will deter carrot fly. Such herbs can be planted in rows between vegetables or as borders around the vegetable patch, as well as among flowers in herbaceous borders and rose gardens. When prepared as a strong infusion they can also be used as plant sprays *(see page 28)*.

The Compost Heap

Fermentation of the compost heap is accelerated by herbs rich in minerals and trace-elements, such as comfrey, dandelion, nettle and yarrow. Fermentation is also assisted by the presence of elder trees, particularly the humus beneath the trees, which is very light and fluffy and makes very good topsoil for the garden.

Growing herbs in small spaces

If you do not have a large garden or any garden at all, you can easily grow herbs in containers of various kinds – in window boxes, troughs, old sinks, urns or decorative pots, including strawberry pots – but they do require a little more care than when

COMPANION PLANTING

Fruit and Vegetables	Good Companion	Plants to Avoid
apple trees	chives, garlic, horseradish	
asparagus	basil, tomatoes	
beans	marigold	chives, fennel, garlic, onions
brussel sprouts	chamomile, coriander/cilantro dill, hyssop, mint, rosemary, sage, thyme	garlic, rue
cabbage and cauliflower	celery, chamomile, dill, hyssop, mint, rosemary, sage, thyme, southernwood, wormwood	strawberries
carrots	chives, coriander/cilantro, flax, garlic, onions, rosemary, sage, wormwood	dill in bloom
celery	chives, dill, leeks, onions, tomatoes	
cucumber	chives, marjoram, nasturtium, nettle spray*	
grapes	basil, hyssop	
lettuce	marigold	
parsnips	garlic	
potatoes	asparagus, horseradish, marigold	rosemary
radishes	nasturtium	hyssop
strawberries	borage, sage	garlic
tomatoes	basil, chives, dill, marigold, parsley	fennel, rosemary
courgettes/zucchini	nasturtium	

grown in open ground. Container-grown herbs are prone both to waterlogging from overwatering and to drying out, particularly in dry weather when they will need lots of attention. They need to be fed regularly and the soil kept just moist all the time. Herbs in containers tend to grow better on balconies and windowsills than indoors, as they get more light and air. They can also be placed on porches and patios, providing there is enough shelter and light – most herbs need a minimum of 5-6 hours sunlight each day.

Terracotta pots and herbs make very attractive partners, though you will need to make sure they are frost-proof or be prepared to take them inside for the winter. In fact, bringing potted herbs indoors in winter is a means of providing yourself with fresh herbs throughout the changing seasons.

In a large outdoor container you can either use garden loam or a loam-based compost. In a smaller pot you can use lighter compost which will need to be replenished each year. Make sure there is proper drainage in your pot before filling it with compost – there need to be holes in the base covered with crocks.

When planting up pots or window boxes, use small herb plants or rooted cuttings and do not be tempted to cram too many plants together in one container as they will fast outgrow their space. Avoid large vigorously growing herbs such as angelica, borage, comfrey, lovage and horseradish. If you want to grow rather invasive herbs like mint, yarrow and lemon balm, the variegated varieties tend to be less fast-growing and so are best. Strawberry pots are pots with holes in the sides and these are excellent for creeping, trailing herbs such as wild strawberry, creeping thyme, pennyroyal and mint. Otherwise, invasive herbs such as mint can be planted in containers and sunk in the ground to contain and restrict their growth.

INSECT REPELLENT HERBS

Insect	Repellent Herbs
ants	marjoram, mint, rue
aphid	basil, chives, coriander/cilantro, elder, nasturtium, tansy
beetles	catmint/catnip, flax, lavender, mint, nasturtium, rosemary, wormwood
black fly	nettle spray*, thyme,
cabbage moth	coriander/cilantro, dill
cabbage worm	chamomile, coriander/cilantro
carrot fly	coriander/cilantro, rosemary, sage, wormwood
caterpillars	elder, mint
fleas	fennel, rosemary, rue
flies	basil, lavender, rue
mice	catmint/catnip, mint,
mosquitos	basil, elder, feverfew, garlic
moths	bay, chamomile, feverfew, lavender

*Nettle spray – Cut nettles and fill a bucket or container of some sort. Cover with water, put lid on and leave to ferment. Fermenting generally takes a few weeks, but they can be left until needed. Strain and spray as insect repellent and plant food.

STRAWBERRY POT

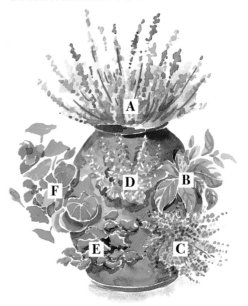

Key to plants:

A	Lavender	**D**	Pennyroyal
B	Basil	**E**	Parsley
C	Thyme	**F**	Nasturtium

Growing herbs in patios or paving

Many herbs look very attractive planted in gaps between stones in patios, paths or paving stones, between bricks or in gravel. Low creeping aromatic herbs are most suitable and are delightful to walk on or by as they release their scents when bruised or brushed against.

If you are laying a path or patio you could either leave random gaps for herbs or design a more symmetrical pattern, the easiest of which is alternate paving stones and herb beds. If your path or patio is already in place, try removing chipped or crumbling corners of the stones or bricks. Squeeze in a little fresh loam and plant your small herb. Suitable plants include chamomile, creeping thyme, marjoram and pennyroyal.

GROWING HERBS

Medicinal herbs consist of a mixture of annuals, biennials, perennials, shrubs and even trees. Annual herbs include basil, borage, German chamomile, coriander/cilantro, dill and marigold, and these can easily be grown from seed. Once grown they may self-seed fairly freely and seedlings can be transplanted to their preferred site in the garden in springtime. Biennials take two summers to come into flower, usually producing an attractive rosette of leaves in the first year. They include angelica, burdock, evening primrose and mullein, all of which also self-seed freely. Herbaceous perennials continue from one year to the next, dying down in autumn and reappearing in spring the following year. They can mostly be grown from seed, but may be easier to grow from other methods of propagation such as root division, or planting cuttings or offsets. Many common herbs can be bought in nurseries or garden

BRICK PATH HERB GARDEN

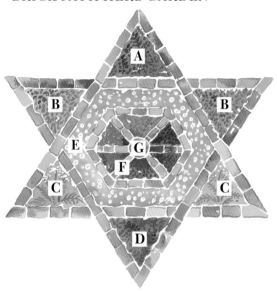

Key to Plants

A	Pennyroyal	**D**	Thyme
B	Corsican Mint	**E**	Chamomile
C	Yarrow	**F**	Thymes
		G	Fennel

PATIO HERB GARDEN

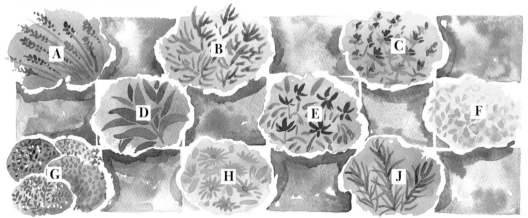

Key to plants

A	Lavender	**D**	Sage	**G**	Thyme
B	Wormwood	**E**	Borage	**H**	Marigold
C	Hyssop	**F**	Oregano	**J**	Rosemary

centres and more unusual herbs can be found in specialist herb nurseries (see page 149). Pot herbs can be planted at most times of the year, except when the ground is frozen or covered with snow, and provided they are healthy they will establish themselves with very little trouble. Always ensure that you choose strong healthy-looking plants, free from disease or insects, and avoid straggly plants and those whose roots are escaping from the bottom of the pot. Make sure the plants are clearly labelled to avoid confusion later. If you want your herb garden to look established after only a short time, buy two or three of each herb to plant in groups. Some fast-growing perennials may have to be moved once they grow and need more space. Try to avoid planting new pot herbs in dry, hot weather. Keep the plants well watered in dry weather until they are firmly established.

Sowing seeds

Herb seeds can be bought from specialist suppliers (*see page* 149) or collected from the previous year's plants. For early plants sow seeds in pots or seed trays in a greenhouse or propagator in early spring (*see below*).

When the seedlings are large enough to handle, you can thin them or transplant them to pots to encourage growth. Once they have become sturdy little plants they are ready to plant outdoors in early summer. Alternatively, you can sow seeds directly into warmer soil in later spring or early summer once all sign of winter frosts has gone. Cover the seeds with soil, the depth of which can be measured by multiplying the diameter of the seeds two to three times.

Growing herbs from seed is both rewarding and fascinating, particularly if you are using seed that you have collected

SOWING SEEDS

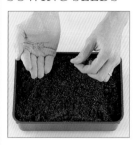

1 Fill a seed tray with well-watered compost. Sprinkle seeds over the surface.

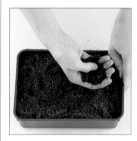

2 Cover the seeds with a thin layer of compost or fine sand. Water and label.

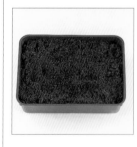

3 Cover with glass. Remove the glass when the seedlings begin to brush against it.

yourself. You may often find that your own seeds germinate more successfully than bought ones, particularly if they are fresh and sown the moment they are ripe and ready to drop. They can be sown in trays and left in a greenhouse or cold frame covered with a piece of glass or polythene until they germinate. This may not happen until the following spring, so you'll need to be fairly patient.

Many variegated types of herbs and decorative coloured herbs such as purple and golden sages will not come true when grown from seed and therefore need to be propagated by other methods, such as root cuttings or root division.

Many herbs self-seed freely if their seed heads are left alone – these include chamomile, coriander/cilantro, dill, elecampane, fennel, lady's mantle, marigold and motherwort. The seeds will then germinate when conditions are right and will grow into strong, healthy plants which can generally be moved easily if – as is likely – they do not fall exactly where you want them in the garden.

Root division

Herbs that form good clumps are excellent candidates for root division, and in fact herbs such as bergamot, catmint, comfrey, valerian and yarrow need to be divided every three to four years into smaller clumps for best results. Root division is best done in the autumn or early spring. First cut back the top growth and dig up the entire plant with a fork. Carefully divide the clump into several pieces with your hands, making sure that each piece retains a good system of roots, and replant in the part of the garden that you have chosen. If the clump is too solid to divide with your hands, you will need to use a garden fork. Dig the fork into the middle of the clump and lever it about, forcing the clump to separate.

Taking cuttings

Taking cuttings from established plants is an easy way to propagate herbs and can be extremely rewarding. Softwood, semi-ripe and hardwood cuttings can all be taken, depending on the plant. Softwood cuttings are generally successful with most herbaceous perennials, while semi-ripe and hardwood cuttings are suitable for shrubs and small trees.

Softwood cuttings

These are best taken in spring and early summer from healthy-looking plants. Once you have inserted them around the edge of your pot or tray, spray the cuttings with water using a plant spray and cover with a propagator lid, a sheet of polythene or an inflated plastic bag to retain the moisture. Roots develop quickly on softwood cuttings, generally within three to six weeks, but it can take just a few days in warm conditions. Root development stimulates leaf growth, so you will know roots are formed when you see tiny new leaves shooting at the growing tip. Once the root system has established itself, the cutting can be gently lifted and potted up in an individual pot or planted in a nursery bed. Cuttings are generally best kept in pots in a sheltered area or in a greenhouse or plastic tunnel during the first winter, and planted out in spring.

Semi-ripe cuttings

These are taken in summer when stems are harder, as they ripen at the base but are still flexible. Side-shoots are taken off new growth, torn away from the main stem, leaving them with a little heel of older wood. Once inserted in pots or trays and watered in, they are also best covered with plastic to retain moisture, but it is not absolutely vital as they are more resilient than softwood cuttings. However, these cuttings take considerably longer to root, so keep them in pots in a cold frame or a sheltered area of the garden, out of direct sunlight, until growth starts the following spring.

Hardwood cuttings

These are taken in autumn, once the plant is dormant, from shrubby herbs or trees such as bay, hawthorn, rosemary, southernwood

TAKING CUTTINGS

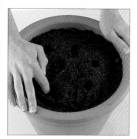

1 Fill a pot with compost and make small holes round the edge with your finger or a stick or dibber.

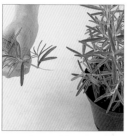

2 Choose several shoots and break them off, making sure that a small heel is left at the bottom.

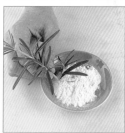

3 Strip off the lower leaves of the cuttings and dip the ends into hormone rooting powder.

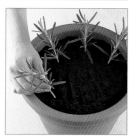

4 Plant the cuttings in the holes and firm the soil around them.

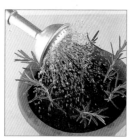

5 Water well and leave. When new growth is seen at the tips of the cuttings, transfer to individual pots.

and witch hazel. Take a side-shoot up to 30cm (12in) long from the current year's growth, remove the lower leaves and insert half its length in a mixture of compost and light soil in a sheltered position in the garden. Firm the soil around the cutting and water it well. Leave in position for about a year until a good root system has developed.

Root cuttings or offsets

This is the ideal method of propagation for herbs that have running roots or that send up side-shoots around the main plant, such as chamomile, comfrey, elecampane, mint, pennyroyal and yarrow. Cut the spreading roots or runners from the parent plant at the end of summer or early autumn. Cut the root into small pieces approximately 5cm (2in) long and put them flat on top of a compost with a little sand in a seed tray. Cover with a plastic sheet and leave in a cold frame, greenhouse, plastic tunnel or sheltered part of the garden. Once new shoots appear, remove the plastic and plant out.

Layering

Low-growing and shrubby herbs such as lavender, periwinkle, sage and thyme can be propagated by layering. Take a low-growing branch and fix it with a peg or a stone so that it is in contact with the soil. If you nick the underside of the branch, it will root more readily. Once a root has developed you can separate the newly formed plant using garden scissors, dig it up and replant.

Mounding

Spreading herbs such as chamomile can be partially covered with soil, thus bringing many different parts of the plant in contact with the soil so that, once rooted, new plants can be separated off the main one.

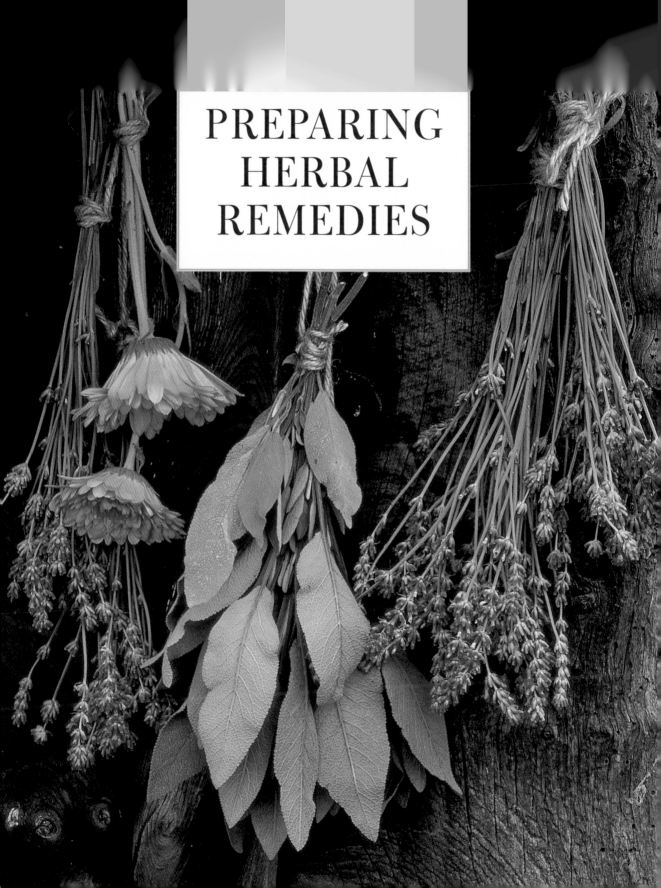

PREPARING
HERBAL
REMEDIES

When harvesting herb plants, it is important to establish first which part of the plant you need – the leaves, flowers, root, rhizome or seeds – and then you can work out when that part is best harvested.

Generally speaking, the aromatic leaves of herbs such as basil, lemon balm, mint, sage and thyme are best harvested when the flowers are about to open, as it is then that the essential oil content is highest. Flowers and flowering tops such as agrimony, goldenrod, hyssop, St John's wort, skullcap and yarrow are best picked just as they are about to burst into bloom. Herbs are best collected on a dry day once the dew has dried. Use a flat basket in order to avoid bruising or crushing leaves or flowers. Herbs for use fresh in the kitchen – such as basil, chives, fennel, mint, parsley, rosemary and sage – can be picked throughout the growing season . Since the growing time for herbs is relatively short, some extra ones could be harvested for drying or freezing to last through the winter months. Particularly valuable are those herbs which could be useful for treating winter colds and coughs, such as ground ivy, hyssop, mullein and thyme, and for fevers, such as chamomile, elderflowers and yarrow.

Seeds such as dill and fennel need to be caught when ripe, before they drop. When harvesting them, you can cut off the whole flower head, tie it up in muslin or a paper bag with string or a rubber band and hang it upside down in a well-ventilated dry room. As the flower head dries, the seeds will conveniently drop into the bag. Store the seeds in envelopes, foil or small boxes with well-fitting lids and label clearly with the herb name and collection date.

Roots and rhizomes of herbs such as burdock, dandelion, elecampane and valerian are best harvested when the aerial parts (flowers and leaves) have died down in autumn or before growing recommences in springtime, as this is the time when they are richest in stored food.

In general, when harvesting, choose plants that look as healthy and vibrant as possible, free from disease and infestation. Make sure they are growing well away from areas that have been sprayed or polluted by traffic, industry or animals. Pick only the amount that you need at any one time, as herbs will easily spoil and be wasted. Harvest just a few leaves and flowers from each plant so as not to threaten the health or survival of any one plant.

DRYING HERBS

The object of the drying process is to reduce or eliminate the moisture in the herb quickly before it starts to die so that it retains its therapeutic properties while being stored for a few months.

When harvesting flowers and leaves for storage pick them in the morning before the heat of the day reaches its peak, but make sure they are dry from rain or dew. Pick them by hand unless stalks, such as those of agrimony or yarrow, are very tough, in which case you will need scissors. Pick gently, taking care not to bruise the plant.

When lifting roots, dig them up with a garden fork, trying not to puncture the outer skin. Wash the soil off the roots and cut off any leaves left. Chop the roots into sections or slices to speed drying and lay them out to dry. When peeling bark, as from witch hazel, it is best to remove the bark from whole branches that have been pruned, rather than shaving it off branches that are still growing, as this may not do the tree much good.

Drying needs to occur as quickly as possible. Shade, air and an even temperature are all vital. Herbs can be dried in shaded, warm but well-ventilated rooms, garden sheds or barns that are free from moisture and condensation. Try to avoid the bathroom and utility room and damp sheds or garages, as the herbs will not dry properly in a steamy, damp atmosphere.

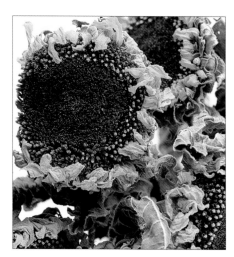

You can loosely tie aerial parts of herbs in small bunches by their stems, and hang them from a beam or a hook indoors. In warm, dry weather, you can hang up bunches of herbs out of doors, out of direct sunlight. This may be rather an unpredictable way to dry herbs, as the temperature varies so much through 24 hours. You will probably get more reliable results if you spread sprigs of herbs, seed or pieces of bark or root evenly over either a tray, wire netting, box lid, fruit tray, sheet of paper or muslin, or, better still, a drying frame. These can be made fairly easily by stretching muslin over a wooden frame, and are excellent for drying as they allow free circulation of air. Spread out the herbs so there is plenty of space between them and turn them frequently – once or twice on the first day and once daily after that. Large-leaved herbs will dry more quickly if the leaves are stripped from their fleshy stems and the stems discarded. A steady temperature of about 27-32°C (80-90°F) is ideal – such as above an Aga or Rayburn stove, in an airing cupboard, or in a slow plate-warming oven with the door left open to allow water to evaporate and air to circulate. If the atmosphere is too cold – below 22°C (72°F) – the plants will reabsorb moisture from the air and deteriorate. Always dry herbs separately – never mix one species with another.

Before storing herbs, check that they are properly dry by seeing if they are brittle and snap easily between the fingers and thumb. If stored before they are completely dry herbs will reabsorb moisture from the atmosphere and deteriorate. It takes between three and seven days for most herbs to dry. Before storing, remove stalks and twigs from aerial parts of plants, and break roots, rhizomes and barks into small pieces.

Herbs are best stored in air-tight dark containers. Clear glass jars are fine if they are kept in the dark, as exposure to light will cause deterioration of medicinal constituents of the herbs. Never store in plastic as it encourages condensation. Make sure to label the herbs by name and the date harvested. Store seeds in packets in the refridgerator or in airtight jars.

Some herbs are ideal for freezing, particularly those with soft leaves such as comfrey, fennel, lemon balm, marjoram, mint and parsley. Pick the leaves or flowers, wash them, shake or pat them dry and place them in small, sealed plastic bags in the freezer. Most herbs will keep until the next growing season if stored in this way.

HERBAL REMEDIES

Herbal remedies can be prepared for both internal and external use. Preparation and use range from the simple application of the leaf to the skin – as for a nettle sting – or the addition of the chopped herb to food – mint on lamb, for example – to the preparation of a tincture for internal use or as the basis of an ointment or salve. Medicinal plants can be prepared for both internal and external use. Which method you choose is really a matter of personal preference. There are no hard and fast rules, although hot decoctions and infusions are particularly recommended for fevers, catarrh and skin problems, and cool ones for kidney and bladder problems. Normal dosage is one cup three times a day for chronic problems and six times a day or more often in cases of acute illness.

INTERNAL USE

Taken internally, raw or as an infusion or tincture, the therapeutic constituents of the herbs enter the bloodstream via the digestive tract.

Decoctions

Decoctions are similar to infusions but involve a boiling process to break down the hard woody parts of plants – bark, seeds and roots – to allow the therapeutic compounds to be absorbed by the water. Either buy these already powdered or be prepared to break them up in a pestle and mortar (much easier if the roots are fresh) or grind them in a coffee grinder.

To make a decoction, you will need:
25g (1oz) dried herbs or 50g (2oz) fresh herbs
650ml (2¾ cups) cold water

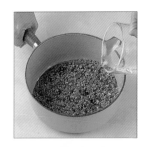

1 Place herbs in a stainless steel or enamelled pan (not aluminium) and cover with water.

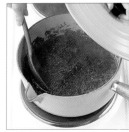

2 Bring to boil, cover and simmer for 10-15 minutes.

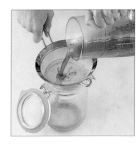

3 Take off heat, strain, and either store or drink immediately.

Infusions

The most widely known and used herbal preparation is a tisane or tea made with the leaves, stems and flowers of dried or fresh herbs. Traditionally, herbs such as chamomile, elderflower, lemon balm and peppermint have been used in teas, but many herbs can be prepared this way. They are mainly prepared with boiling water except in the case of herbs with a high percentage of mucilage, such as comfrey and marsh mallow root, which must be made up with cold water and left to infuse for 10-12 hours. If poured into an airtight container, infusions can be stored for up to two days in a refrigerator.

You can adjust the standard recipe to taste

and, if it is too bitter, combine the herbs required with more palatable herbs such as lemon balm or peppermint, or sweeten them with honey.

Infusions are usually taken hot, particularly for fevers and colds; they are taken lukewarm or cold, however, for problems associated with the kidneys and urinary tract such as cystitis and urethritis.

To make an infusion, you will need:
25g (1oz) dried herbs (leaves/stems/ flowers) or 50g (2oz) fresh herbs
600ml (2½ cups) boiling water

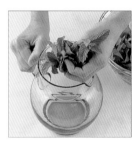

1 Warm the jug or pot with warm water then add the herbs.

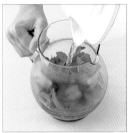

2 Boil water. When it is just off the boil, add it to the herbs. Cover the container and leave to infuse for 10 minutes.

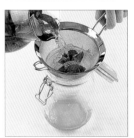

3 Strain and and either drink immediately or store.

Syrups

Syrups often make herbal remedies more attractive to children. Dosage is two teaspoons for children, three or four times a day for chronic problems and six to eight times a day in acute illness. If you have no decoction or infusion prepared, one teaspoonful herbs can be mixed with honey and given to children (one teaspoonful three times a day for chronic problems and one teaspoonful every two hours in acute illness).

To make herbal syrup (recipe one):
650g (24oz) mixture of thin honey and unrefined sugar (ratio 1:1)
600ml (2½ cups) double strength infusion/decoction

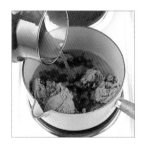

1 Heat infusion or decoction with honey in a stainless steel or enamelled pan.

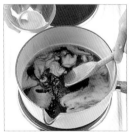

2 Stir mixture as it starts to thicken and skim off scum from surface.

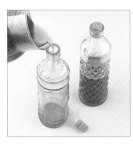

3 Leave to cool before pouring into a cork-topped bottle. Drink immediately, or store in a refrigerator.

To make herbal syrup (recipe two):
600ml (20floz) boiling water

**1.25kg (2½lb) thin honey or unrefined
   sugar**
Herbal tincture of choice (*see below*)

Make syrup base by pouring boiling water
over sugar and stir over low heat until sugar
dissolves and solution starts to boil. Remove
from heat and add herbal tincture in a ratio
of one to three. This can be stored in an
airtight container indefinitely.

Tinctures

Tinctures are alcoholic extracts of herbs
which are complex to prepare but which can
be kept for two years or more and need only
be taken in small amounts. They can be
taken internally, used to make ointments and
lotions, and added to bath water.

The herb, fresh or dried, is macerated
(soaked for softening) in a mixture of water
and alcohol according to ratios laid down in
a herbal pharmacopoeia. The ratio varies
from plant to plant, depending on the
constituents the plant contains which need
to be extracted by the water and alcohol
mixture. Some tinctures can be made with
neat cider vinegar, producing herbal
vinegars such as garlic or rosemary vinegar
for culinary use, or raspberry vinegar for
treating children's coughs and sore throats.
For children (and adults) who require a
sweeter taste, you can prepare tinctures
using equal parts of water and glycerol. For
more watery fresh herbs, such as borage, use
80 per cent glycerol. Herbs suited to this
method include catmint, elderflowers and
nettles.

The standard recipe is one part dried
herb to five parts fluid, or one part fresh herb
to two parts fluid. Brandy or vodka, which
are 60-70 per cent proof (45 per cent
alcohol), provide a good alcohol solution
and can be used in the following recipe.
Normal dosage for chronic problems is one
teaspoonful for adults or 10 drops to half a
teaspoonful for children, three times a day;
for acute illness the dosage can be doubled.
Mix with a little water, juice or herbal tea. For
gargles, use half to one teaspoonful in a
cupful of water two to three times a day or
every two hours for acute conditions.

To make a tincture:
200g (7oz) dried chamomile flowers
**1 litre (4⅓ cups) 45 per cent alcohol
   solution (*see above*)**

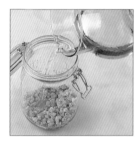

1 Pour solution
over herbs in jar.
Seal with airtight
lid. Leave to
macerate away
from light for two
weeks. Shake daily.

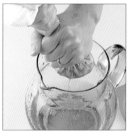

2 Press the
mixture through a
muslin bag into a
jug.

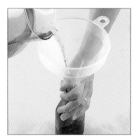

3 Pour into a dark,
labelled bottle and
store in a cool
place.

Tablets and capsules

Tablets and capsules can either be bought from herb suppliers and health food shops or made at home by filling gelatine capsules (available from specialist suppliers) with powdered herbs. Standard capsule sizes are O which holds around 0.35g powder and OO which holds around 0.5g. Standard dosage is three capsules size O or two capsules size OO, three times a day. Capsules should not be used for bitter herbs which need to be tasted to trigger reflexes in the rest of the digestive system.

Suppositories

Suppositories inserted into the rectum are quickly absorbed into the bloodstream. Moulds can be bought from specialist shops or made from aluminium foil. They can be kept refridgerated for up to three months.

To make five suppositories:
5 tsp dried herbs
10 tsps (⅔ cups) cocoa butter, melted

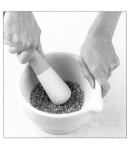

1 Use a pestle and mortar to crush the dried herbs to powder.

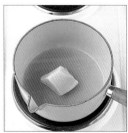

2 Melt cocoa butter in a saucepan.

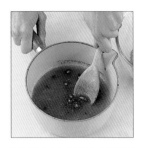

3 Remove pan from heat and mix in powdered herbs.

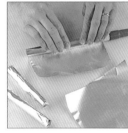

4 Make moulds by rollling tinfoil around a thick pen (approximately 1cm (⅜in) diameter).

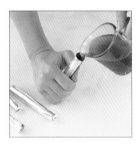

5 Pour mixture into moulds to a depth of 2cm (¾in). Twist the end of the tinfoil to secure the mould and leave to cool.

EXTERNAL USE

Infusions and decoctions can be used in eyebaths, gargles and lotions. Dosage is two to three times daily for chronic problems and every two hours in acute cases.

There are several external pathways by which herbal constituents can be introduced to the bloodstream – through the skin, through the nasal passages via inhalation, and through the conjunctiva of the eye. Infusions and decoctions can be added to bathwater, and salves, creams, poultices and compresses can all be applied to relieve pain and irritation. Dilute essential oils can be used similarly.

Herbal baths

Warm water opens the skin's pores so that when herb infusions or decoctions or essential oils are added to a bath, the plant constituents are quickly absorbed, while the volatile oils are inhaled through the nose and mouth into the lungs and thus into the bloodstream. The oils also affect the nerve receptors in the nose which carry messages to the brain. For luxurious relaxation, add chamomile and lavender, or for a touch of stimulation, add rosemary.

Add a few drops of essential oil (see below) to bathwater – always dilute oil first for babies, children and those with sensitive skin. Add around 600ml (20fl oz) strong herb infusions (i.e., double dose infusions). Soak in bath for 15 to 30 minutes for maximum effect.

Hand and foot baths

Hand and foot baths are an easy way of introducing herbal constituents to the bloodstream, since hands and feet are both sensitive areas with plenty of nerve endings. The French herbalist Maurice Messegue recommends eight-minute foot baths in the evening and eight-minute hand baths in the morning (four minutes each time for children).

Salves and creams

Salves are made by macerating herbs in oil; creams are made by stirring tinctures, infusions, decoctions or a few drops of essential oil into a base of aqueous (water based) cream, available from pharmacists.

To make salve
450ml (2 cups) olive oil
50g (2oz) beeswax
Herb – fresh or dried

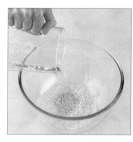

1 Mix oil and beeswax together in a heatproof dish.

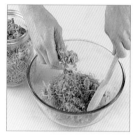

2 Add as much of your chosen herb as the mixture will cover and mix.

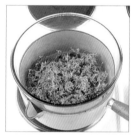

3 Heat gently over a saucepan of boiling water for 2-3 hours.

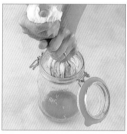

4 Press out through a muslin bag, discard herb and pour the warm oil into a jar. Leave to solidify.

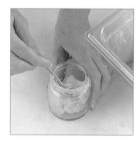

5 The salve may be spooned into small glass containers for easy access. Store in a cool place, or use immediately.

To make chamomile cream:
2-3 drops blue chamomile oil
50g (2oz) aqueous cream

Mix together and smooth into skin. This recipe is good for many types of eczema.

Compresses and Poultices
Both poultices and compresses are applied to areas of pain or swelling. Poultices use the herb itself, while compresses involve some form of extract.

To make a poultice:
Herbs – fresh or dried
Two pieces of gauze
Light cotton bandage

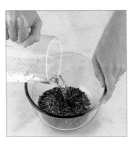

1 If using fresh herbs, bruise using a pestle and mortar. If using dried herbs, add hot water to make a paste.

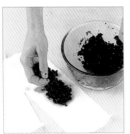

2 Place sufficient herb to cover the affected area between two pieces of gauze.

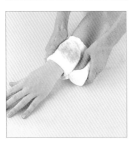

3 Use a light cotton bandage to bind the poultice to the affected area. Keep it warm with a hot water bottle.

To make a compress:
Herbal preparation of your choice – hot or cold infusion or decoction, or water with a few drops of essential oil
Flannel or small towel

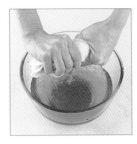

1 Soak cloth in a herbal preparation of your choice. Remove flannel from bowl and wring out the excess liquid.

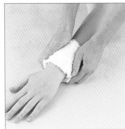

2 Apply to affected area, repeating several times.

Oils

Essential oils cannot be prepared at home because they are extracted from plants by steam distillation, but they can be obtained from health food shops and other stockists (*see page* 149). However, infused oils can be prepared at home, and used for inhalations and external applications, such as massaging inflamed joints, or for neuralgia, bruises or swellings.

To make an infused oil:
1 litre (4⅓ cups) cold-pressed safflower, walnut or almond oil
Fresh or dried herbs (the quantity will depend on the size of jar used – herbs should be sufficient to pack jar)

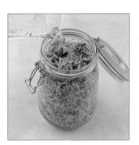

1 Pack a glass jar with a herb and cover with oil. Seal with airtight lid. Leave in a sunny place for two weeks. Shake daily.

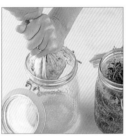

2 Squeeze the oil through a muslin bag into a jar.

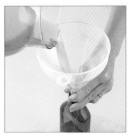

3 Strain and pour into dark-coloured storage bottles.

Liniments

A liniment is a rubbing oil or embrocation used in massaging muscles and ligaments. It may contain stimulating essential oils to increase local circulation so that the herbal constituents quickly reach the affected part when absorbed by the skin. A liniment consists either of extracts of herbs in an oil or alcohol base, or herbal or essential oils and an alcohol tincture of your choice.

To make liniment:
25 drops rosemary essential oil
25 drops lavender oil
10 drops marjoram oil*
1 drop capsicum tincture
50 ml (¼ cup) almond oil

Shake well before use.

* Avoid during pregnancy

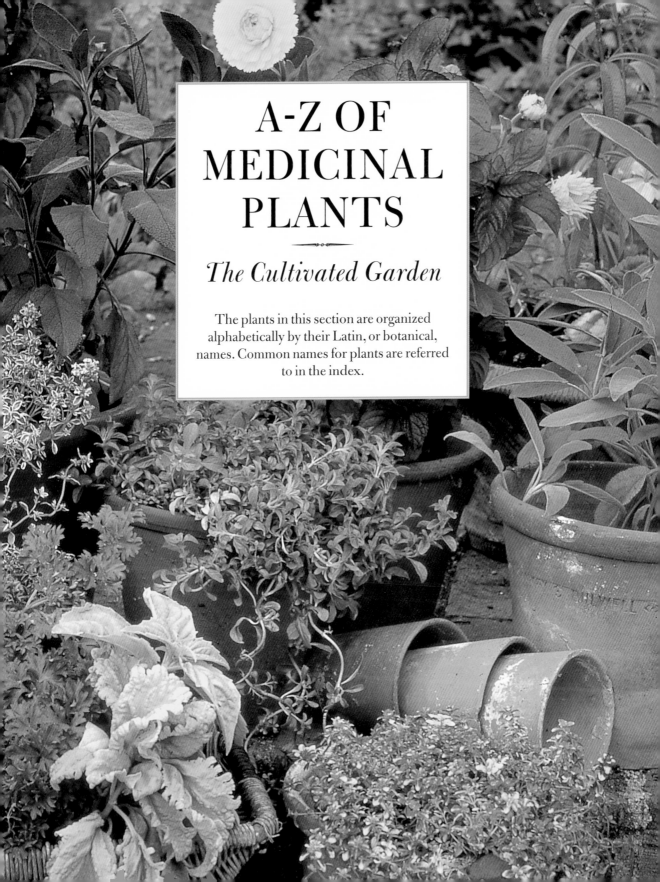

A-Z OF
MEDICINAL
PLANTS

The Cultivated Garden

The plants in this section are organized
alphabetically by their Latin, or botanical,
names. Common names for plants are referred
to in the index.

Achillea millefolium
YARROW

Part used: Leaves and flowers
Contains: Volatile oil, sterols, bitters, tannins, salicylic acid, coumarins

Yarrow is an attractive perennial member of the *compositae* family, with numerous feathery aromatic leaves, hence *millefolium*, Latin for 'a thousand leaves'. With its minute white or pink flowers, it can be found growing wild in hedgerows, lanes and meadows, or on light sandy soils, and it is quite drought resistant. Its extensive superficial roots bind loose soil together and prevent it from being eroded.

Yarrow has been valued as a medicine since at least the times of the ancient Greeks. The generic name *achillea* comes from the legend of Achilles, who healed his companion's battle wounds with yarrow. The plant was still used as a first-aid dressing in the First World War. It has also been considered a sacred plant, imbued with spiritual powers, and used both to protect against evil and as a love charm and in China for divination with the I Ching.

Yarrow is still used as an excellent healing remedy, with its antiseptic, anti-inflammatory and astringent actions and silica to promote tissue repair. Used externally, it will speed healing of cuts and wounds, ulcers and burns and can be applied to varicose veins, haemorrhoids and skin conditions like eczema. Internally yarrow makes a good digestive remedy for diarrhoea, wind, indigestion and inflammatory problems such as gastritis and colitis. It acts to regulate the menstrual cycle and as a tonic to the nervous system. In a hot tea it promotes perspiration and makes a good remedy for fevers as well as colds, flu, catarrh and childhood infections such as measles and chicken pox. It is an excellent circulatory remedy, helping to lower blood pressure and relieve problems such as poor circulation and varicose veins.

How to Grow: Propagate by sowing seeds in spring or autumn in well drained soil and full sun. Alternatively, divide the plant in spring or autumn. Grows 15-60cm (6-24in) high and flowers from July to September.

Alchemilla vulgaris
LADY'S MANTLE

Part used: Root, leaves and flowers
Contains: Salicylic acid, tannins, bitters, saponins, volatile oils, phytosterols

Lady's mantle is an attractive hardy perennial with distinctive pale-green leaves and tiny, lacy green-yellow flowers, providing decorative ground cover for many weeks.

The medieval alchemists, whose interest in the plant is reflected in its generic name *alchemilla*, called the little dew-like drops of water that exude from the leaves 'water from heaven'.

The medieval Christians dedicated lady's mantle to the Virgin Mary, as the leaves were thought to resemble her cloak. It was highly valued as a wound healer to staunch bleeding and the dew-drops were considered a vital aid to women's beauty.

Lady's mantle, as its name suggests, is an excellent internal astringent and anti-inflammatory remedy for women; for heavy periods, painful or irregular periods, to aid contractions during childbirth and to enhance recovery afterwards. It is helpful when treating genito-urinary infections, fibroids and pelvic inflammatory disease. It also benefits the digestive tract, and is useful for diarrhoea and inflammatory problems such as gastritis, colitis or gastro-enteritis and the urinary system, as it has diuretic properties. Externally, lady's mantle makes an excellent douche for vaginal infections, a skin lotion for rashes, cuts and abrasions and a gargle for sore throats.

NB: Avoid during pregnancy

How to Grow: Propagate by sowing seeds in early summer in seed trays. Keep moist but do not cover. Plant out when large enough to handle. Alternatively, divide clumps in early spring or autumn. Self-seeds freely. Prefers moist and fertile soil and tolerates sun or shade. Grows 15-45cm (6-18in) high. Flowers from June to September.

Related plants
Alchemilla arvensis: Parsley piert – a smaller plant common in dry soil, in fields and waste ground, even walls. Excellent for urinary problems, particularly stones and gravel.

Allium sativum

GARLIC

Part used: Bulb
Contains: Volatile oil, mucilage, germanium, glucokinins, vitamins

This powerful-smelling perennial is a member of the lily family and makes an excellent companion plant in fruit and vegetable gardens and under roses to keep aphids away.

Garlic is a wonderful medicine, valued for thousands of years. The ancient Egyptians used it for its energy-giving properties around 1500 BC and the Greeks and Romans, including Dioscorides and Galen, considered it a panacea and elixir of youth. Ayurvedic doctors in the 1st century AD in India prescribed garlic for heart disease, while for centuries it has been used for warding off not only a whole host of infections but other evils such as vampires, witches, demons and the evil eye.

Garlic is truly an excellent remedy for infections, having antibacterial, antiviral, antiparasitic and antifungal properties. Internally, it exerts its effects throughout the digestive, respiratory and urinary systems, disinfecting as it goes, enhancing immunity and remedying coughs and colds, stomach and bowel infections, as well as cystitis. It also acts as a decongestant, good for catarrh and hay fever, and an expectorant, useful when treating coughs and asthma. Garlic is a wonderful medicine for the heart and circulation, lowering raised blood pressure and harmful cholesterol levels and reducing the tendency to blood clotting, thereby helping to reduce heart attacks and strokes. Its antioxidant properties help the body withstand the ageing process, and at the same time garlic acts as an invigorating tonic – a veritable 'elixir of life'.

How to Grow: Propagate by planting cloves of garlic in early spring or late autumn in well drained, moderately rich soil and full sun. Harvest late summer when the plant dies down, leave to dry outside for a few days, then tie in bunches to hang or store in a cool dry place. Grows 15-30cm (6-12in) high.

Allium schoenoprasum
CHIVES

Part used: Leaves
Contains: Essential oil (containing sulphur)

Attractive hardy perennials, chives can look very decorative in clumps in the herb garden or as edging plants, with their purple pom-pom flowers and bright green leaves. With their strong anti-fungal and insecticidal properties, they make good companion plants for vegetables, fruit and flowers prone to aphids.

Chives are the smallest member of the onion family, but probably the one most widely grown in herb gardens. They may well have been known by the ancient Greeks and Romans as they grow wild in Greece and Italy and were cultivated in Britain by the Middle Ages. Chives were included in King Charlemagne's recommendations for planting, written in 812, and grown by Parkinson in his garden in the 17th century.

Taken internally, chives have valuable medicinal use, although they have not been formally employed as a medicine. Added to soups, salads and as a garnish, fresh chives will serve to enhance the immune system and provide valuable antiseptic properties, having antibacterial, antiviral and antifungal actions. They have a warming and stimulating effect on the digestion, enhancing digestion and absorption. Their vitamin C and iron content help combat infection as well as anaemia.

How to Grow: Propagate by sowing seeds in April/May or dividing clumps in spring or autumn. Plant in fertile, moisture-retentive soil, full sun or light shade. Grows 15-40cm (6-16in) high and flowers throughout the summer. Remove the flowers to stimulate maximum leaf growth. Divide clumps every 2-3 years.

Althea officinalis
MARSH MALLOW

Part used: Roots, leaves and flowers.
Contains: Mucilage, tannins, asparagin, polysaccharide, sugars

Marsh mallow is a lovely stately perennial with velvety leaves and soft pink flowers, often found growing wild in damp salty marshes as its name suggests, by the seaside. Butterflies love it.

Marsh mallow was grown by the Romans

CHIVES (*Allium schoenprasum*)

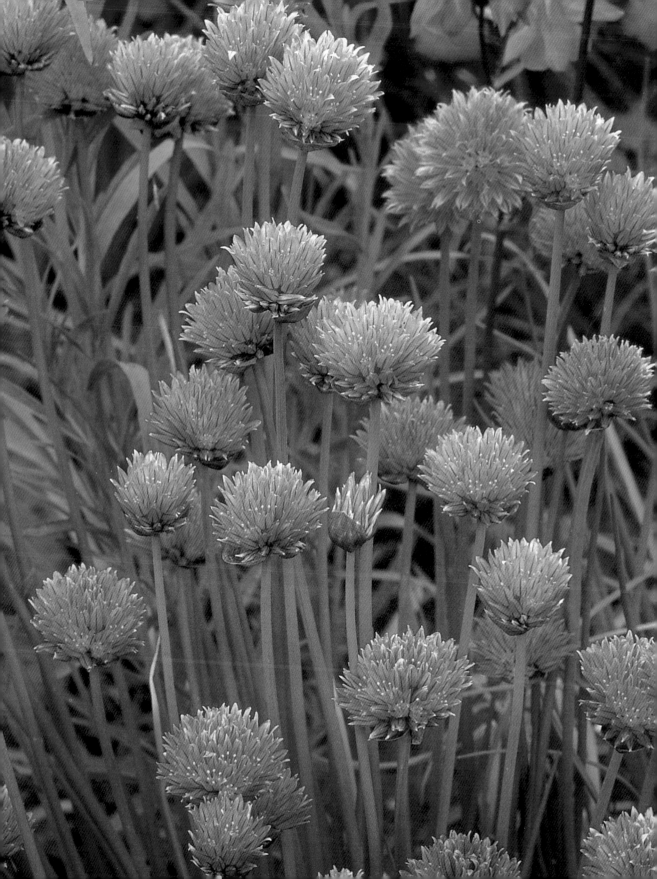

who enjoyed the root as a vegetable, and the tender leaves and young tops were eaten by the ancient Greeks. Aristophanes spoke of eating mallow shoots instead of wheat. Followers of Pythagorus considered mallows sacred, as their flowers always turned towards the sun.

The abundance of mucilage, particularly in the root, makes marsh mallow the most soothing of medicines, wonderful for all kinds of irritation and inflammation, internal or external. It soothes harsh dry coughs, sore throats, asthma, croup and bronchitis, relieves digestive problems such as heartburn, colitis and gastritis and acts as a diuretic, relieving cystitis and an irritable bladder. Marsh mallow leaves can be rubbed onto insect bites, scalds and burns, sunburn and skin rashes. A warm poultice will help draw splinters out, while a gargle can be used for sore throats and inflamed gums.

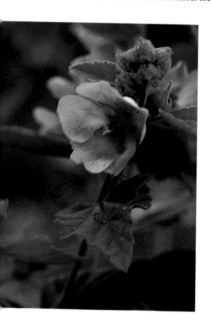

How to Grow: To propagate, sow seeds in damp soil in late spring or in trays in autumn and leave outside over the winter. Alternatively, divide roots in spring or autumn. Grows 0.6-1.2m (2-4ft) high, and flowers from July to September from its second year.

Anemone pulsatilla
PASQUE FLOWER

Part used: Dried leaves and flowers
Contains: Glycoside, ranunculin (poisonous in fresh plant), which yields anemonin, tannins, saponins, resin

The hardy perennial pasque flower, with its silky purple flowers and silvery hairs like a halo, followed by feathery seed heads, is one of the most beautiful wild flowers of temperate climates. Delicate looking, it is remarkably resilient, flowering in early spring but often in very wintery weather.

It is said that pasque flowers were originally called passe flowers, from the French *passe-fleur*, meaning that it surpassed all other flowers in beauty. In 1597 Gerard renamed it pasque flower as it came into flower at Easter (or *Pâques* in French) and was popular for dyeing Easter eggs green.

Pasque flower is an excellent relaxant as well as a tonic to the nervous system. Able to relieve spasm and reduce pain, it is useful, taken internally, for colic, period pain, headaches, asthma and neuralgia. It is recommended for those suffering from nervous exhaustion, depression or insomnia, particularly those who tend to become irritable and weepy. Because of its astringent and bactericidal action on the mucous membranes, pasque flower also makes a good remedy for colds, catarrh, coughs, ear and eye problems.

How to Grow: Pasque flower is found growing wild on limestone or chalk, in dry grassy places. It reaches about 30cm (1ft) high. It grows well in well drained alkaline soil and full sun and can be propagated by seed sown in early summer and barely covered with soil. Germination may be slow.

Anethum graveolens

DILL

Part used: Leaves, seeds
Contains: Volatile oil, flavonoids, coumarins

Dill is an aromatic annual with feathery leaves, originating in the Mediterranean. The leaves are delicious with meat and fish dishes, lending an aniseed taste, while the seeds are traditionally used as a pickling spice.

The tranquilising properties of dill have been known since the days of the ancient Greeks and Romans. Its name is said to come from the Saxon word *dilla*, 'to lull', due to the plant's ability to relax babies into a sleep. In medieval times, however, dill was known as an ingredient of love potions and as protection against witchcraft.

The leaves and seeds contain a volatile oil that, taken internally, has a relaxant effect on muscles. It releases tension and spasm in the digestive tract, relieving colic and wind, indigestion, nausea, and constipation as well as diarrhoea. It is an important ingredient in the famous 'gripe water', used by generations of mothers to relieve babies' colic. Dill can also be used for harsh dry coughs and asthma, and to relieve period pain and regulate menstruation. It has traditionally been used to ease childbirth and enhance milk supply in feeding mothers.

How to Grow: Propagate by sowing seeds in spring and again in midsummer, in rich, well drained soil and full sun. It likes a sheltered position. Grow well away from fennel as they cross-pollinate easily.

Angelica archangelica

ANGELICA

Part used: Roots, leaves, stem, seeds
Contains: Essential oil, coumarins, resins, sugars, starch

This tall, architectural biennial, largest of the Umbelliferae family, has large leaves and hollow stalks that make a tasty addition to salads when young, much like celery. Candied stalks have long been used to decorate cakes and puddings and the seeds used in making vermouth and chartreuse.

Angelica was highly valued by our ancestors as an antidote to poisons and a remedy for infectious diseases as well as to protect against spells of witches and evil spirits. It is linked in Christian mythology with the Annunciation and it was believed that its healing properties were revealed to a monk during an epidemic of the plague by an angel – hence its Latin name.

Angelica has a sweet pungent taste and a warming effect throughout the body, and taken internally it is of benefit for people with poor circulation who feel the cold in winter. It makes an excellent remedy for a weak digestion that causes nausea, indigestion, wind and colic. It has antibacterial and antifungal properties and a cleansing effect generally, helping to detoxify the body and enhance immunity. As a warming expectorant it can be used for coughs, asthma and catarrh, and as a hot tea it will bring down fevers. It helps to regulate the menstrual cycle and relieve period pain and pre-menstrual syndrome. It has an overall strengthening effect and acts as a tonic to the nervous system.

How to Grow: Propagate by sowing seeds in autumn as the seeds benefit from exposure to frosts, or pre-chill in the refridgerator for a few weeks if sowing in spring. Prefers rich, moist soil and light shade. Grows up to 1.80m (6ft) tall. Flowers July to August. If all but one flower are removed it will live for several years.

Related plants
A. atropurpurea: American angelica – popular among the Shakers as a flavouring agent and medicine similar to A. archangelica.
Angelica polymorpha var. *sinensis*: Chinese angelica – a wonderful tonic for women and used for a wide range of gynaecological problems.

Apium graveolens
WILD CELERY

Part used: Root, seeds
Contains: Volatile oils, apiol, sulphur

Wild celery is an aromatic biennial member of the Umbelliferae family. It has a fleshy, bulbous root, and is the original celery from which the vegetable we use today was cultivated. From Roman times until the 17th century there was only the wild celery to impart that distinctive pungent flavour to soups, vegetable dishes and stews. It can be found growing wild in or around ponds and ditches, and in marshy ground.

Wild celery has been used not only as a food but also for its medicinal benefits since Roman times. It was popular in the Middle Ages for its ability to relieve aches and pains, to remedy the digestion, and calm the nerves. It was highly valued as an aperient, to promote the flow of digestive juices and

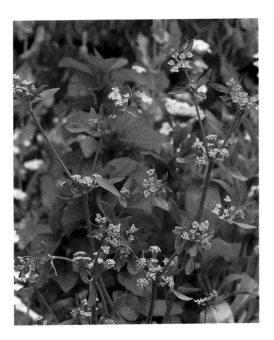

ensure regular working of the bowels. It was also praised as a remedy for overweight and for fluid retention.

Wild celery has a similar action to parsley, both containing apiol, an antiseptic constituent with a particular affinity for the urinary system. Taken internally, it has a diuretic effect and so relieves fluid retention and cystitis, and helps to eliminate toxins from the system. Celery makes an excellent remedy for arthritis and rheumatism as well as gout. It also acts as a tonic to the digestive tract, and has an uplifting effect upon the nervous system.

How to Grow: Propagate by sowing seeds in March/April in a greenhouse in trays and plant out when large enough and there is no danger of frost. Prefers deep, damp, well-manured soil and not too much sun. Grows 30-60cm (1-2ft) high and flowers from late summer to early winter.

Artemisia abrotanum
SOUTHERNWOOD

Part used: Leaves and flowers
Contains: Essential oil – mainly absinthol, bitters

Southernwood is a handsome semi-evergreen perennial shrub, with grey-green feathery and highly aromatic leaves which were traditionally used as an insect repellent and to keep moths out of clothes, and as nosegays to protect against contagion. It is a good companion plant in the vegetable garden and orchard as its insecticidal properties deter aphids and cabbage butterflies.

The Greeks and Romans placed southernwood under mattresses for its aphrodisiac powers. In Elizabethan England, it was regarded as a remedy against the plague and was placed near prisoners in the dock to protect the court from gaol fever. It was used as a flavouring for ale before the introduction of hops.

Taken internally, the bitter taste of southernwood stimulates the flow of digestive juices and promotes appetite and improves digestion and liver function. It removes both threadworms and round-worms from the bowel. It has an affinity for the female reproductive system, promoting menstruation and increasing efficiency of contractions during childbirth. Southernwoood has antiseptic properties and a tonic effect on the nervous system.

NB: Avoid during pregnancy.

How to Grow: Propagate by taking young green cuttings in summer or hardwood heeled cuttings in late summer or autumn.

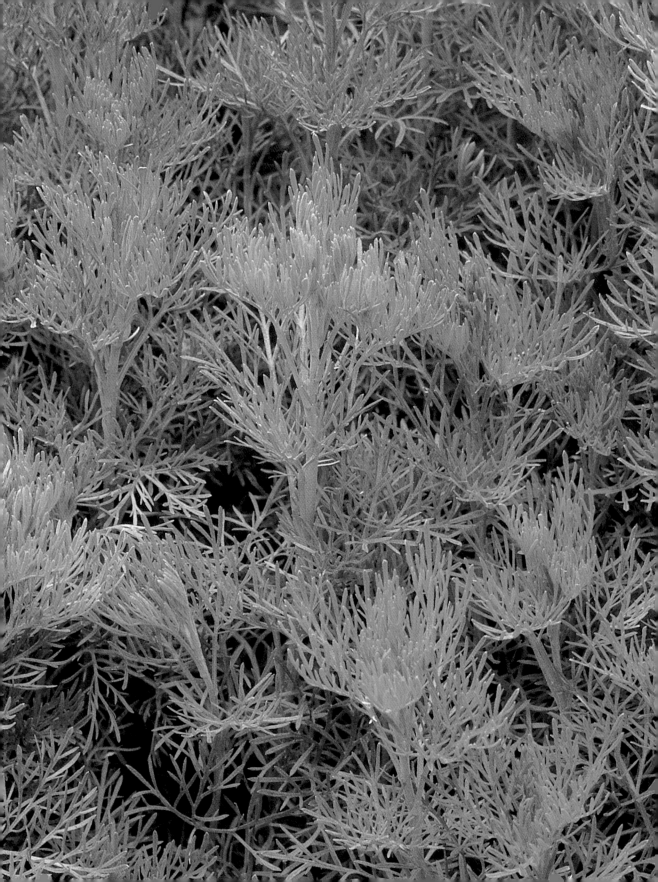

Prefers light well-drained soil and full sun. Needs trimming in mid-spring to prevent it from growing straggly. Grows 0.9-1.5m (3-5ft) high and rarely flowers in temperate climates so it is hard to collect seed.

Artemisia absinthium

WORMWOOD

Part used: Leaves and flowers
Contains: Volatile oil, bitters, tannins, carotene, vitamin C

Wormwood is a lovely bushy perennial plant, popular in gardens for its silky silver-grey leaves which are highly aromatic. It makes a good companion plant as it deters pests in the garden, particularly moths and ants. It can be found growing wild in dry stony places, even out of walls, particularly in the Mediterannean.

For centuries wormwood has been a major ingredient in bitter aperitifs and wines such as vermouth. Wormwood's medicinal use is recorded in the Ebers Papyrus written in Egypt around 3500 years ago. The classic Greek herbals recommended it to promote digestion and as a powerful tonic and aphrodisiac. Like the other artemisias, it is named after the Greek goddess, Artemis, who took care of women, particularly during childbirth, and it has been used throughout history to enhance contractions and promote the birth.

One of the most bitter herbs, wormwood, if taken internally, stimulates the appetite and promotes digestion and liver function. It is excellent for weak, sluggish digestion, liver problems and worms and to cleanse toxins from the system, particularly for those feeling debilitated or when recovering from illness. It enhances the immune system and taken hot brings down fevers and relieves colds and flu, catarrh, food poisoning and skin problems. It is a good remedy for irregular or painful periods and helps to promote contractions in childbirth.

NB. Avoid during pregnancy.

How to Grow: Propagate by taking cuttings in summer or sow tiny seeds in a tray, water lightly but do not cover with soil. Best to cover the tray with glass until seed germinates. Plant out in autumn or spring, in well-drained, fertile soil and full sun. Grows 0.6-1.2m (2-4ft) high and flowers in July to August. Self-seeds easily.

Related plants
A. vulgaris: Mugwort – often found growing wild. Has similar uses to wormwood and southernwood – excellent bitter tonic, woman's remedy and antiseptic.
A. annua: Sweet wormwood – used in Chinese medicine and becoming well known for its antimalarial properties.

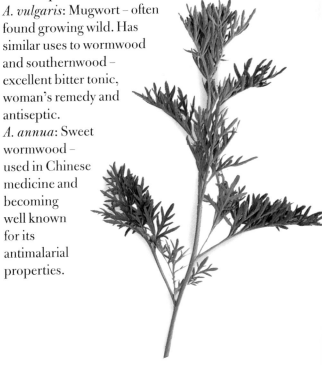

SOUTHERNWOOD (*Artemisia abrotanum*)

Avena sativa

WILD OATS

Part used: Whole plant and seed
Contains: Saponins, alkaloids, sterol, flavonoids, starch, protein, fats, minerals, vitamin B

Wild oats are annual tufted grasses, often found growing wild, having escaped from cultivated fields. They are wonderfully nutritious, full of protein, calcium,

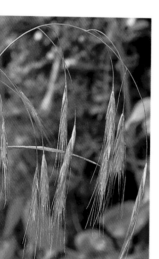

magnesium, silica, iron and vitamins which help make good bones and strong teeth and are vital to a healthy nervous system. They make an excellent energy-giving food and body builder.

Taken internally, oats make an excellent tonic to the nervous system, supporting the body during times of stress and relieving depression, anxiety, tension and nervous exhaustion. They are well worth taking when withdrawing from tranquilisers and antidepressants. Oats in the diet can significantly lower blood cholesterol and help combat cardiovascular problems. They are a good remedy for constipation and help to prevent bowel cancer by removing toxins from the bowel. Since they lower blood sugar they make a very useful food for diabetics. They also have the ability to regulate hormones in the body, notably oestrogen. Used externally, oatmeal makes a good facial scrub and soothing remedy for inflamed skin conditions.

How to Grow: Propagate by sowing seed in spring in well-drained fertile soil and full sun. Grows up to 90cm (3ft) tall. Plants are harvested in summer before they open fully, and are threshed to separate the grain.

Calendula officinalis

MARIGOLD

Part used: Flowers
Contains: Carotenoids, resin, essential oil, flavonoids, sterols, bitters, saponins, mucilage

The bright and cheerful marigold is a popular annual plant of old-fashioned cottage gardens. Both the leaves and flowers make an excellent addition to soups and salads, while in the garden the marigold is a good companion plant, deterring infestation of its neighbours. Marigolds have long been popular as a cosmetic herb and a dye to colour a variety of foods including soups and conserves.

The Romans used marigolds to bring down fevers and applied the flowers to warts. In medieval times they remedied intestinal problems, liver complaints and insect and snake bites. Gerard and Culpeper recommended them to comfort the heart and lift the spirits, for inflammation of the eyes and for 'trembling of the heart'. They were said to protect against evil influences and disease including the plague. The Shakers used them for gangrene.

Marigolds are astringent and antiseptic, and taken internally are excellent for enhancing the immune system and treating a wide variety of infections, including flu and herpes viruses; fungal infections such as candida; and pelvic and bowel infections

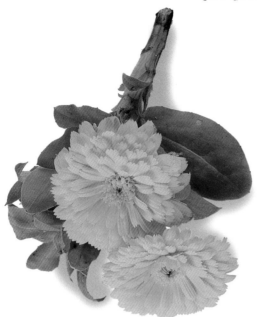

including enteritis and worms. In the digestive system marigolds relieve irritation, inflammation and diarrhoea and enhance digestion and absorption as well as liver function. Taken hot, marigolds bring down fevers, improve blood and lymphatic circulation and help the body to throw off toxins. They help regulate menstruation and clear congestion in the reproductive tract that contributes to pain, excessive bleeding, tumours and cysts. Their oestrogenic properties are very valuable during the menopause. Externally, marigolds are famous as a first-aid remedy for cuts and abrasions, sores and ulcers, burns and cold sores, to staunch bleeding, reduce infection and speed healing.

NB: Avoid during pregnancy.

How to Grow: Propagate by sowing seeds in spring or autumn in moist, medium-rich soil and full sun. Grows 30-50cm (12-20in) tall and flowers from June to September or first frosts. Deadhead regularly to ensure continued flowering.

Carduus/Cnicus benedictus

HOLY THISTLE

Part used: Root, leaves, flowers and seeds
Contains: Alkaloids, mucilage, tannin, bitters, essential oil, flavonoids

This hairy, prickly annual thistle grows such a profusion of leaves and flowers that it is often hardly able to keep upright under its own weight. The fresh green leaves used to be eaten with bread and butter for breakfast. When found growing wild they are said to indicate fertile ground and they make an excellent addition to the compost heap.

The apothecaries of the 16th and 17th centuries held holy thistle in high esteem, particularly as a cure for the plague and to strengthen the nerves. Gerard grew it in his garden and Culpeper recommended it for giddiness and vertigo, liver and gallbladder problems, to cleanse the blood and clear the skin.

Taken internally, holy thistle is used today as a tonic to the nervous system, to aid

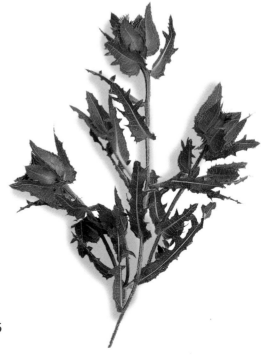

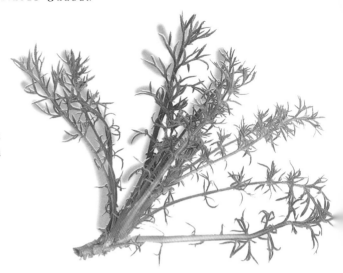

digestion and absorption, and to treat the liver. It makes an excellent remedy for indigestion, diarrhoea, wind, poor appetite, headaches and lethargy and can be taken to restore energy after illness or when feeling run down. It strengthens the immune system and has an antimicrobial action and has been shown to have anti-tumour activity. Taken hot, it reduces fevers and catarrhal congestion, and improves circulation. It is a wonderful woman's remedy, increasing milk production, reducing heavy periods and relieving headaches and period pain.

How to Grow: Propagate by sowing seed in spring or autumn in loose fertile soil with full sun. Holy thistle grows to about 60cm (2ft) high and flowers in July and August.

Chamomilla recutita
CHAMOMILE

Matricaria chamomilla
GERMAN CHAMOMILE

Anthemis nobilis/
Chamamaelum nobile
ROMAN CHAMOMILE

Part used: Flowers
Contains: Volatile oil, flavonoids, coumarins, plant acids, fatty acids, cyanogenic glycosides, salicylate derivatives, choline, tannin

There are two kinds of chamomile used medicinally, the annual German chamomile and the perennial Roman chamomile. Their properties are almost identical but German chamomile is often preferred as it tastes less bitter. Roman chamomile is often used in the

planting of aromatic lawns, paths and arbours, releasing its heady fragrance as it is walked on. German chamomile grows wild in cornfields and all over the Mediterranean.

Chamomile was recommended by Dioscorides as a cure for fevers as early as 900 BC and was known to the ancient Egyptians who praised it for its ability to cure malaria and dedicated it to the sun god, Ra, for its power to reduce fevers. It was one of the nine sacred herbs of the Saxons who used it as a calming remedy and to treat stomach problems. In the Middle Ages it was frequently strewn in the insanitary halls of castles and great houses to keep infection at bay as well as to disguise the smell.

Taken internally, chamomile is an excellent relaxant, calming anxiety and nervousness, and is well-suited to tense, stressed people who tend to be over-sensitive and very active. It can be used for treating all stress-related problems, particularly those affecting the digestion, such as acid indigestion, colic, abdominal pain, peptic ulcers, wind, diarrhoea and constipation. It is well known for calming restless babies prone to colic, teething and sleeping problems, as well as overactive, irritable children. It induces restful sleep and also has pain-relieving properties – it can be taken for headaches, neuralgia, toothache, aches and pains of flu, arthritis and gout. It relieves period pain and pre-menstrual headaches and eases contractions during childbirth. Chamomile has antibacterial and antifungal properties and makes a good remedy for thrush. It also acts as a natural antihistamine, reducing allergic symptoms in hay fever, eczema and asthma. Externally it has an antiseptic and anti-inflammatory action, excellent for healing sores, burns and scalds and a whole range of skin disorders.

How to Grow: Propagate German chamomile by sowing seeds in spring or autumn in well-drained, preferably chalky soil; do not cover the seeds but water them in. Grows up to 45cm (1ft 6in) tall and flowers through the summer. Self-seeds freely. Likes a sunny position.

Propagate Roman chamomile by sowing seeds in spring, taking cuttings in summer or dividing the plant in spring or autumn. Do not cover the seeds with soil as they need light to germinate. Prefers light, fertile, well-drained soil and full sun. Flowers through the summer.

Cichorium intybus
CHICORY

Part used: Root, leaves and flowers
Contains: Root – inulin, bitters, taraxasterol, cichoriin tannins, alkaloids. Leaves and flowers – inulin, fructose, esculetin, resin, cichoriin

Chicory is an attractive herbaceous perennial, a relative of the dandelion, with pretty, bright blue daisy flowers, which open only from 8am till noon. It has a large taproot which is specially cultivated for a substitute or an additive to coffee, which helps to counteract the stimulating effects of caffeine. The young leaves, often forced and blanched, are excellent in salads.

Chicory was highly valued as a medicine by the ancient Egyptians and is mentioned on a papyrus dating back 4000 years. The ancient Greeks and Romans knew it as a vegetable, and referred to chicory coffee as 'liver's friend' for its benefits to the liver and gallbladder. Parkinson called it a 'fine cleansing jovial plant'.

Like the dandelion, chicory is an excellent bitter herb which, when taken internally, increases appetite and promotes digestion and absorption. It stimulates the function of the liver and gallbladder and can be used for mild constipation, conditions associated with a sluggish liver such as headaches,

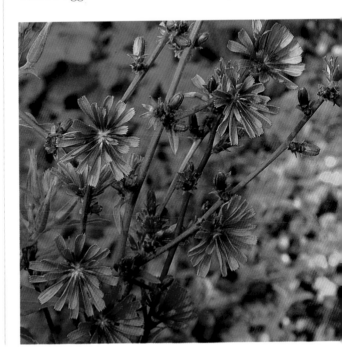

irritability and skin problems, as well as gallstones. Its diuretic action helps relieve fluid retention and clear toxins from the system, and its antibacterial effect is useful in combating infection. It is helpful to diabetics as it reduces blood sugar and it also has a regulatory effect upon the heart.

How to Grow: Chicory can be found growing wild, to a height of 0.9-1.5m (3-5ft) and flowering from June to October. Propogate by sowing seeds in late spring in rich soil and full sun.

Cimicifuga racemosa
BLACK COHOSH

Part used: Dried roots and rhizomes
Contains: Triterpene glycosides, tannins, volatile oil, resin, salicylates, ranunculin (poisonous in fresh plant) which yields anemonin

Black cohosh is a tall elegant perennial found growing wild in shady woods in North America and Canada. Its small white feathery flowers on graceful slender spikes used to be called fairy candles. Its Latin name comes from *cimex*, 'a bug', and *fugare*, 'to flee', as the smell of the plant was renowned for driving away insects.

Black cohosh was a popular plant among the North American Indian women, as a remedy for uterine problems and to aid childbirth. Once recognised as a medicine by orthodox doctors it was valued for its benefit in treating whooping cough, bronchitis, heart problems, rheumatism, neuralgia and

menstrual problems. It was also considered an excellent antidote to poisons, particularly of rattlesnake bites.

Black cohosh, with its powerful painkilling properties, is excellent, taken internally, for relieving muscle and nerve pain, as well as arthritis, headaches, uterine pain, breast pain and contractions during childbirth. The salicylates have anti-inflammatory properties and also help pain relief. Black cohosh relaxes muscles, easing cramp and colic, muscle tension, asthma and whooping cough. By dilating the arteries, black cohosh can reduce high blood pressure, and it also benefits the heart, normalising its action. Its oestrogenic properties can be helpful through the menopause.

NB: Do not take in large doses. Avoid during early pregnancy.

How to Grow: To propagate, sow bought seeds (as it does not set seed properly in Great Britain) in spring or autumn in good, moist, fertile and well-drained soil. Will grow in sun or shade, and reaches a height of 1.2-2.4m (4-8ft) flowering from July to September.

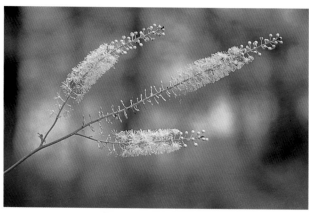

Coriandrum sativum

CORIANDER/CILANTRO

Part used: Leaves and flowers, seeds
Contains: Volatile oil, malic acid, tannin

Coriander is a highly aromatic annual member of the *Umbelliferae* family, with attractive leaves like parsley which are delicious in salads and soups. The seeds are one of the oldest recorded spices, referred to both in ancient Sanskrit texts and in the Old Testament, where they are mentioned as one of the bitter Passover herbs.

Coriander is an ancient medicine, used by the ancient Greeks and Egyptians and by the Romans who brought it to England from where it travelled to America, to be one of the first spices grown there. It was valued for its stimulating digestive and aphrodisiac powers and, according to Chinese medicine, it was able to confer longevity and even immortality on those who ate it.

Taken internally, coriander is an excellent digestive, enhancing the appetite and improving digestion and absorption of nutrients. It strengthens the nerves and is a good remedy for stress-related digestive disorders, such as gastritis and peptic ulcers. It has a cooling effect useful for fevers

and hot inflammatory problems, such as cystitis, conjunctivitis, sore throats, arthritis and skin rashes. Its relaxant effect relieves colic and period pain and explains its ancient use during childbirth.

How to Grow: Propagate by sowing seeds in fertile, well-drained soil and full sun in early spring and at regular intervals through the summer, or under glass in autumn. Keep well watered in dry weather to promote growth of larger lower leaves.

Cynara scolymus

GLOBE ARTICHOKE

Part used: Flower heads, leaves, root
Contains: Bitters, flavonoids, inulin, taraxasterol, volatile oil, sugars

The globe artichoke is an impressive hardy perennial, and a favourite ornamental as well as edible plant, with its silvery leaves and large grey-blue thistle-like flowers. The flower heads are popular as a vegetable, especially in Mediterranean countries.

Globe artichoke is one of the oldest cultivated vegetables, valued by the ancient Greeks and Romans and introduced into Britain in the early 16th century as a vegetable and ornamental plant in monastery gardens. It was used as a medicine by the medieval Arab physicians, particularly to treat the liver and sluggish digestion.

Taken internally, the bitters in artichoke leaves stimulate bile secretion from the liver and gall bladder and the flow of digestive

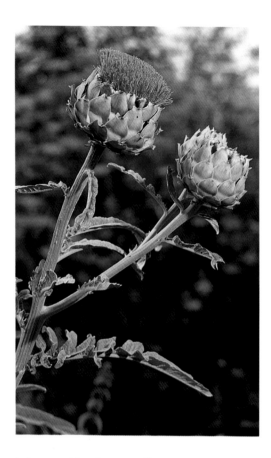

Echinacea augustifolia/Echinacea purpurea/Echinacea pallida

PURPLE CONE FLOWER

Part used: Root and rhizome
Contains: Essential oil, polyacetylenes, glycoside, isobutyalklamines, resin, sesquiterpene

Purple cone flower, also known commonly as echinacea, is a lovely perennial plant with pink-purple, daisy-like flowers, found growing wild in many parts of North America. The generic name comes from the Greek word *echinos*, meaning 'hedgehog', because of its black shiny seed heads. It makes an interesting and colourful addition to a herb garden and flower border; in fact *E. purpurea* has been grown in European gardens for nearly 300 years.

Echinacea was discovered by the North American Indians and became one of their most important medicines. The Cheyenne chewed the root to quench their thirst, particularly useful when doing the strenuous 'Sun Dance', as it stimulates the flow of saliva. Others used it as a local anaesthetic to relieve toothache, headaches, stomach pain and back ache. It was regarded as an antidote to snake bites and excellent for infections such as coughs and colds, measles and mumps, boils and abscesses.

Today echinacea makes an excellent internal remedy for all kinds of infections and is becoming increasingly popular. Taken every two hours it will help the immune system fight off sore throats, colds and flu, chest infections and glandular fever to name a few. It has antibacterial, antiviral and

PURPLE CONE FLOWER
(*Echinacea augustifolia*)

juices, making it an excellent remedy for weak digestion, heartburn, nausea, poor appetite, liver insufficiency and jaundice. In Europe particularly, artichoke is used to lower cholesterol and triglyceride levels, and to treat arteriosclerosis. Its diuretic properties help to relieve fluid retention as well as urinary infections.

How to Grow: Propagate by sowing seed or planting suckers growing from the root stock (retaining a piece of the parent plant) in rich moist soil in late spring or early summer. Likes full sun and plenty of water. Grows 0.9-1.75m (3-5ft) and produces flowers in mid to late summer. Replace every 5 years to ensure good flower crop.

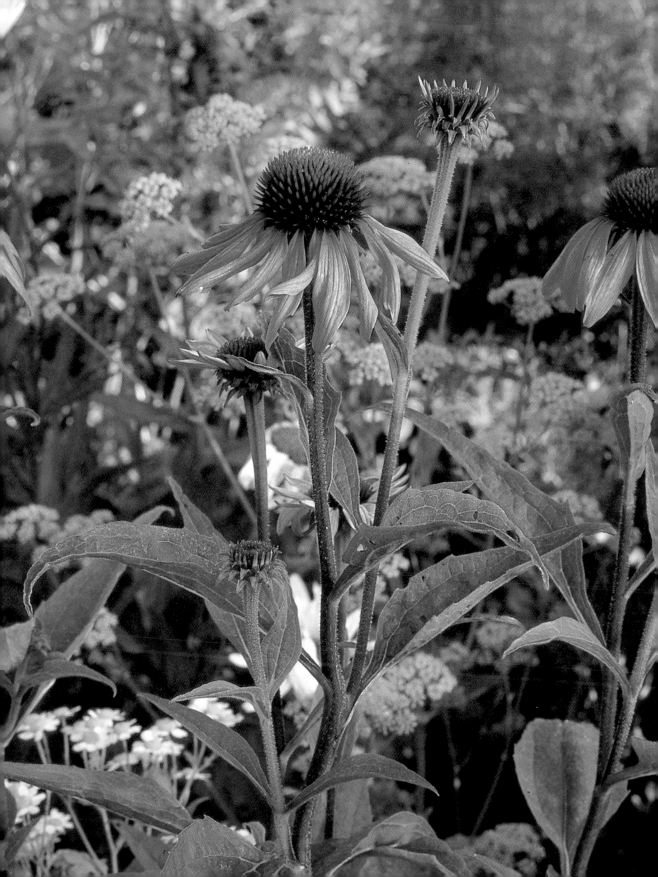

antifungal actions, as well as anti-allergenic properties. Its benefits in the treatment of human immuno-deficiency virus (HIV) and AIDS are currently being investigated. Echinacea also has anti-inflammatory properties, excellent for relieving arthritis and gout and problems such as pelvic inflammatory disease. It enhances the circulation and when taken hot will bring down a fever.

How to Grow: Propagate by sowing seeds or dividing the roots in spring or autumn. Seeds germinate better if sown on the surface of a sandy soil mix in an open cold frame in January although *E. purpurea* can be sown directly in the garden. Prefers moderately rich and well-drained soil and full sun, although *E. purpurea* enjoys dappled shade. Grows 0.6-1.2m (2-4ft) high and flowers June to September. Roots can be harvested 3 to 4 years after planting seed, two years after root division.

Erica/Calluna vulgaris/Erica tetralix /Erica cinerea

HEATHER

Part used: Flowering tops
Contains: Flavonoid glycosides, carotene, citric and fumaric acids, arbutin, tannins, volatile oil, resin, alkaloids

Heather is a popular evergreen sub-shrub with pretty little pinky-purple flowers, found growing wild on acidic, sandy soils or peat bogs, in woodland, moors and hillsides. Many horticultural cultivars are grown for decorating the garden. Heather is loved by bees and butterflies, and looks beautiful in dense masses.

The generic name erica comes from the Greek word meaning 'to break', as heather has long been regarded as an excellent cure for expelling or dissolving urinary stones and gravel. It was used in baths for easing joint and muscle pain, and taken for urinary infections and to ease sleep.

Today, heather makes a useful urinary antiseptic when taken internally due to the arbutin it contains, and can be taken for cystitis, urethritis and prostatitis. It has a mild diuretic action, reducing fluid retention and hastening elimination of toxins via the kidneys. It therefore makes a good cleansing remedy for gout

and arthritis as well as skin problems such as acne. It has a mildly sedative action and can ease anxiety, muscle tension and insomnia.

How to Grow: Propagate by taking cuttings in August and inserting them into a mixture of peat and sand. Alternatively, sow seed in autumn in peaty soil and cover with sand. They may take as long as 20 years to germinate! Heather can also be layered in spring. It likes acidic sandy soil and full sun, or semi-shade. Grows up to 60cm (2ft) tall and flowers from July to September.

Eupatorium purpureum

JOE PYE WEED

Part used: Rhizome and roots
Contains: Flavonoids, volatile oil, resin

Joe Pye weed is a very handsome North American perennial with a mass of pink-purple flowers, often found in moist woodland and meadows and by streams. Its Latin name comes from the ancient Greek King of Pontus, Mithradatus Eupator, one of the first to use eupatoriums as medicines, while its common name is after the famous Joe Pye, a New England medicine man who cured fevers and typhus from decoctions of this plant.

Joe Pye weed was a popular remedy among the North American Indians. Women would bathe sick children in a tea made from the roots, and the early settlers learnt to use it for gout, rheumatism, neuralgia, fluid retention and urinary problems, particularly stones and gravel – it was often known as gravel root for this reason.

Today, Joe Pye weed is still popular as an internal remedy for the urinary system and for treating urinary infections, stones and gravel, as well as inflammation of the prostate gland. It has a toning effect on the reproductive system and can be taken to relieve menstrual pain and pelvic inflammatory disease. Its diuretic action relieves fluid retention and hastens excretion of wastes from the body, making it a good remedy for arthritis and gout.

How to Grow: Propagate by sowing seeds or dividing roots in autumn or spring. Plant in good, moisture-retaining soil, sun or shade. Grows 0.75-3m (2ft 6in-9ft) high and flowers from midsummer to autumn. An excellent plant for damp borders or round a pond.

Related plants
E. perfoliatum: Boneset – a good remedy for fevers
E. cannabinum: Hemp agrimony – stimulates the immune system

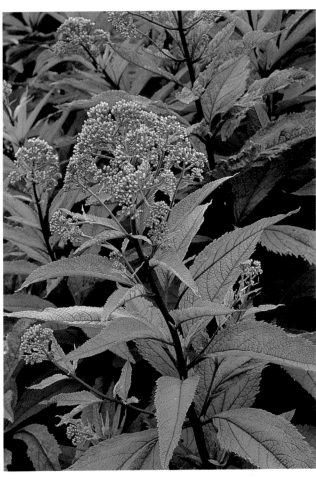

Filipendula ulmaria
MEADOWSWEET

Part used: Leaves and flowers
Contains: Essential oil, salicylates, mucilage, sugar, tannin, citric acid

Meadowsweet is a lovely perennial plant with feathery white almond-scented flowers and attractive red-stalked leaves. It grows in damp water meadows and on river banks, earning its old country name, queen of the meadow. It was once called meadwort, as it was used to flavour mead, and in Chaucer's England it was made into beer.

Meadowsweet was one of the sacred herbs of the Druids and was an important plant of wedding feasts, made into garlands and posies and strewn in churches. It was a favourite chamber herb of Queen Elizabeth I, and loved by Gerard who said its smell 'makes the heart merrie and joyful'. In 1838 salicylic acid was discovered and meadowsweet was found to be a valuable source of the substance we now know as aspirin.

The medicinal action of meadowsweet naturally resembles that of aspirin without the side-effect of stomach irritation. In fact, meadowsweet, taken internally, is actually an excellent remedy for a whole range of digestive disorders, including acidity, gastritis and ulcers. It relieves wind, diarrhoea, enteritis and colic and has an antiseptic as well as anti-inflammatory action. Meadowsweet is a well-known remedy for arthritis and rheumatism. Its diuretic action helps eliminate excess fluid and toxins from the body and its analgesic action soothes pain, not only joint pain but also headaches and neuralgia. It helps to bring down fevers and to bring out rashes in eruptive infections such as measles and chicken pox and thereby speed recovery. The salicylate salts soften deposits in the body such as kidney stones and gravel, as well as atherosclerosis in the arteries.

How to Grow: Propagate by sowing seeds in spring or autumn in moist rich soil and sun/light shade, or in trays of compost under glass. Alternatively divide the roots in spring. Grows 0.9-1.2m (3-4ft) high and flowers in June to September. Keep watered in dry weather.

Foeniculum vulgare
FENNEL

Part used: Seeds, leaves, roots
Contains: Volatile and fixed oil, flavonoids, vitamins and minerals

Fennel is a handsome perennial with blue-green feathery foliage and large umbells of flowers that bear seeds. The whole plant has a delightful aniseed smell and flavour which has been used in the kitchen, in liqueurs and perfumery. The soft growing tips make a delicious garnish for fish dishes and salads; the roots and stalks used to be boiled as a vegetable and the seeds used in bread and cakes. A juicy variety – *F. vulgare* 'Dulce', Sweet or Florence fennel – is grown today as an annual which makes a delicious vegetable.

Fennel was enjoyed as a spice by the ancient Egyptians, Greeks and Chinese. The Egyptians used fennel to treat eye problems and the Greeks valued its detoxifying and diuretic properties to help overcome obesity.

MEADOWSWEET (*Filipendula ulmaria*)

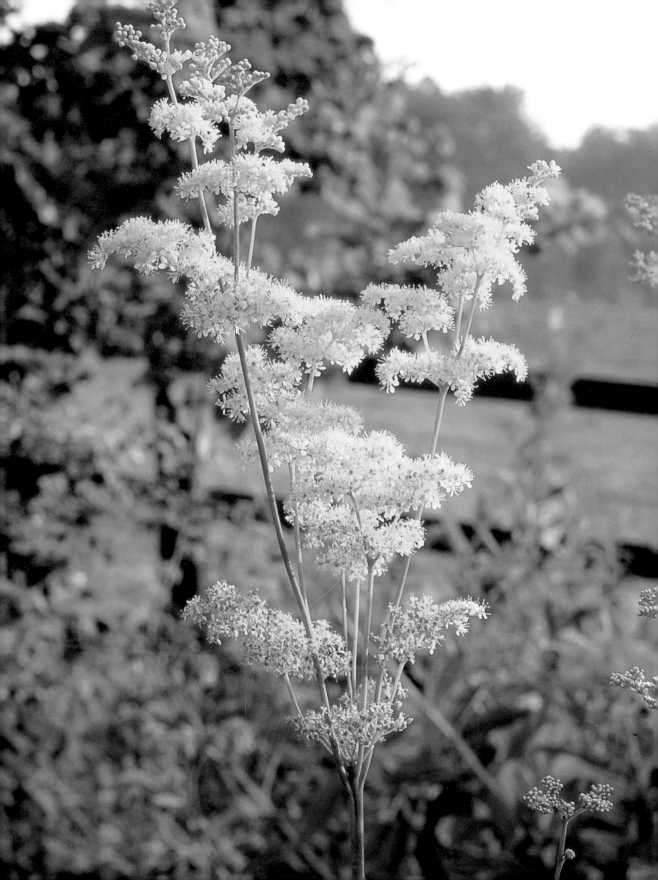

Hippocrates recommended it for stimulating milk flow in nursing mothers. In Greek mythology it was said to give men knowledge, and the Greeks adopted it as their symbol of victory. In the Middle Ages it was said to ward off evil spirits and bad luck.

Taken internally, fennel seeds and roots make an excellent digestive remedy, settling the stomach, relaxing colic and relieving wind, nausea, indigestion and heartburn. The seeds are included in the famous gripe water for babies' colic. As a diuretic, fennel is useful for fluid retention and as a detoxifying remedy, often used for cellulite as well as urinary infections. Its antispasmodic properties help to relieve period pains and its hormone-like action is useful in regulating the menstrual cycle and during menopause. Fennel aids milk production in nursing mothers and, used externally, it makes an excellent lotion for sore eyes.

How to Grow: Propagate by sowing seeds February to May in pots or in well-drained, medium-rich soil and full sun, or divide root in spring or autumn. Fennel likes a warm, sheltered place. Water well in dry weather and cut back to 7cm (3in) above soil in autumn. Self-seeds easily. Replace plants after 3 to 4 years. Do not grow near dill as they readily cross fertilise. Grows 1.5-2m (4-6ft) and flowers from July to October.

Fragaria vesca
WILD STRAWBERRY

Part used Leaves, fruit and root
Contains: Leaves, tannins, flavonoids, fruit, organic acids, vitamin C, mucilage, sugars, pectin

The little wild strawberry plant can be found growing in woods and lanes, and on chalky grassland. It is a hardy perennial and progenitor of the cultivated strawberries we enjoy eating in summer. Its Latin name probably comes from the fragrance of the delicious fruit, and the name strawberry from strayberry as the trailing runners stray all over the ground.

The ancients were familiar with the wild strawberry; both Ovid and Pliny mention it and Virgil considered it a sweet-smelling flower. The fruit was used to treat consumption and in Elizabethan times the leaves were valued as beneficial to the kidneys and the root was used to treat diarrhoea and dysentery, while the delicate smell of the fruit was said to lift the spirits.

Today, strawberry leaves are still valued for their astringent properties. Taken internally, they check bleeding as well as diarrhoea. They make a good gargle for sore throats and mouthwash for bleeding gums. The roots have bitter properties and stimulate the liver and enhance digestion. The fruits are high in vitamin C and can relieve fevers, fluid retention, constipation and gout.

NB. Excessive consumption may lead to allergic reactions.

How to Grow: Propagate by sowing seeds on surface of the soil and keep moist.

Germination may be erratic and slow. Alternatively, plant runners in spring or autumn in good fertile soil. Does not like clay soil very much. Prefers sun or light shade and a sheltered position. Flowers and fruits June/July.

Related plants
F. virginiana – North American wild strawberry with similar properties.
F. moschata – wild strawberry with larger flowers and similar properties.

Fumaria officinalis
FUMITORY

Part used: Leaves and flowers
Contains: Seven alkaloids, bitters, tannins, mucilage, resin, fumeric acid, potassium

Fumitory is a small, unusual annual plant, a member of the poppy family, growing as a weed in fields, banks and gardens in many parts of Europe. Its common name comes from the French *fume de terre* meaning 'smoke of the earth' as its grey-green feathery leaves look like smoke rising from the ground. Pliny said that its juice stimulated such a flow of tears from the eyes that it was as if smoke had got into them. It was also said not to grow from seed but from vapours from the ground.

According to ancient folklore, when fumitory is burned its smoke has the ability to expel evil, and fumitory was included in the medieval St. Gall garden plan for this purpose.

Throughout history it has been praised for its purifying properties and was used for constipation, liver problems and skin eruptions, even leprosy.

Today fumitory is still used for its cleansing properties. Taken internally, it has laxative, diuretic and diaphoretic actions, all hastening elimination of toxins from the body, via the bowels, urine and skin respectively. It acts as a tonic to the liver, and is used not only for digestive problems, but particularly for skin problems of all kinds, including eczema, psoriasis, cradle cap and acne.

How to Grow: Propagate by sowing seeds in spring, in almost any soil, though it particularly likes light, well-drained soils. Spreads very quickly, flowering from May to September and stems reach a length of 15-60cm (6-24in). Self-seeds easily.

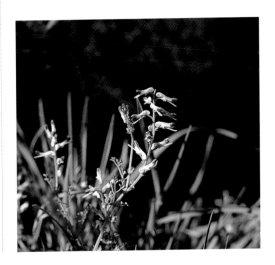

Glycyrrhiza glabra
LIQUORICE

Part used: Roots and runners
Contains: Glycyrrhizin, triterpenoid saponins, flavonoids, bitters, oestrogenic substances, asparagin, volatile oil, coumarins, tannins

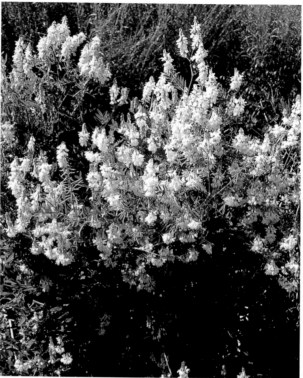

Liquorice is a graceful vetch-like perennial which was introduced to Britain by the Black Friars in the early 16th century. By the 17th century it was grown extensively in Pontefract in Yorkshire for use by brewers and apothecaries. Pontefract cakes can still be found in many confectioners.

Liquorice was well known to the ancient Greeks for treating dropsy and preventing thirst. Its name *glycyrrhiza* comes from Greek words meaning 'a sweet root'. Gerard grew it in his garden as did Parkinson, and Culpeper recommended it, along with rosewater and gum tragacanth, for hoarseness and wheezing. Mixed with cascara it was frequently administered to children as a laxative, and mixed with linseed it was given for troublesome coughs.

Today, liquorice is one of the most popular and versatile of herbal remedies. Taken internally, its anti-inflammatory, anti-allergic and anti-arthritic properties make it an excellent cortisone-like medicine, useful for allergies and inflammatory problems and when weaning off orthodox steroid treatment. It has a long history of use for healing ulcers, and by lowering stomach acid levels it relieves heartburn and indigestion. It soothes irritation and inflammation throughout the digestive tract, and has a beneficial effect on the liver, increasing bile flow and lowering cholesterol. In the respiratory system it has soothing expectorant and anti-inflammatory actions, excellent for irritating coughs, asthma and chest infections. Its oestrogenic properties can be very helpful through the menopause, while the whole plant has the ability to improve resistance to stress.

NB: Long-term use can lead to sodium retention and raise blood pressure.

How to Grow: Propagate by root division in the spring, and plant the root 10cm (4in) deep in plenty of well-drained soil and full sun. Grows up to 1.50m (5ft) high and flowers in midsummer.

Hamamelis virginiana

WITCH HAZEL

Part used: Leaves, bark and twigs
Contains: Tannins, saponins, choline, resins, flavonoids

The witch hazel tree was a favourite remedy of the Native Americans, who dried it and used it as snuff for nosebleeds and mixed it with flax seed to apply to painful swellings and tumours. It has long been known as a household remedy for scalds and burns, to stop bleeding and bruising. The branches used to be valued as divining rods for finding underground water and metals.

The high proportion of tannins in witch hazel makes it excellent as an astringent for

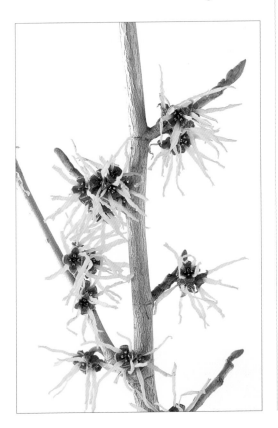

stemming bleeding internally and externally. Traditionally it has been taken internally for heavy periods, colitis, diarrhoea, dysentery and chronic catarrh. Its toning action on muscles throughout the body has been employed to treat uterine prolapse, varicose veins and haemorrhoids, and to tone the uterus after miscarriage or childbirth. Externally, witch hazel makes an excellent lotion for burns, inflammatory skin problems, bruises, sprains, insect bites, inflamed eyes, greasy skins, phlebitis and varicose ulcers.

How to Grow: Propagate by sowing seeds in spring, or layer branches in autumn. Cut out suckers each year and root these to make new plants. Prefers lime-free soils, full sun or light shade. Grows up to 3.90m (13ft) tall and flowers from late autumn to early spring.

Helianthus annuus

SUNFLOWER

Part used: Seeds, flowers, leaves
Contains: Tannins, inulin, levulin, calcium

The splendid sunflower is an annual which derives its name from the fact that it follows the sun's path through the day. It was introduced to Europe from its native Mexico and Peru in the 16th century as it was of enormous economic value. Every part of the plant had some use – the leaves and stalk provided fodder, raw materials for cloth and paper and a substitute for tobacco, the flowers yielded a yellow dye, the seeds produced food and oil, and the pith of the stalk gave a very light substance which was later used to make life-belts.

The sunflower was revered as a symbol of

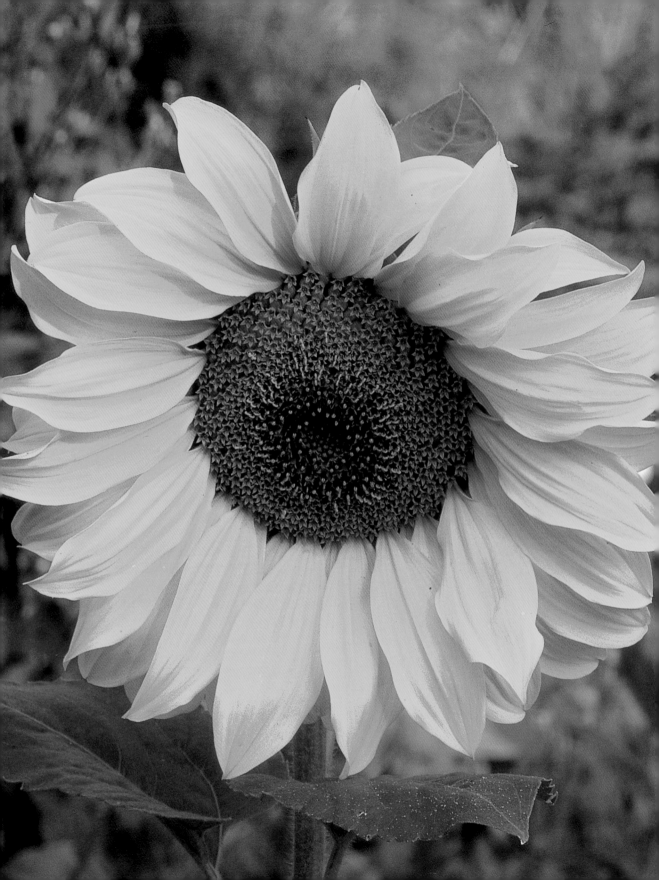

the sun by the Peruvian Incas and the North American Indians. It was carved into the sculptures of their temples and woven in gold into the fabrics of their clothing. The priestesses wore gold crowns carved in the shape of the sunflower.

Sunflowers have been used internally as a folk remedy for sore throats, colds, coughs, and asthma. The seeds were used for intermittent fevers and malaria. Nineteenth-century settlers in America planted sunflowers near their homes as they absorbed the water from damp ground reducing the disease that abounds in damp areas as well as mosquitos that carried malaria. The seeds are highly nutritious, rich in protein, calcium, iron, potassium and magnesium, and have diuretic properties, useful for gout and arthritis. The oil has been found to be useful for treating asthma and externally as a rub for arthritis and rheumatism.

How to Grow: Propagate by sowing seeds in boxes or singly in pots under glass in March and when hardened off plant out in May. Plant at least 90cm (3ft) apart. Sunflowers prefer an open sunny position and plenty of manure but will tolerate any soil. Can grow 0.9-3.6m (3-12ft) high and flowers in August to September.

SUNFLOWER (*Helianthus annuus*)

Humulus lupulus

HOPS

Part used: Strobiles
Contains: Volatile oil, bitter-resin complex (lupulin), tannins, oestrogenic substances, asparagin, trimethylamine

Hops come from the female flowers of a rampant perennial climber which grows wild in hedgerows and is cultivated commercially for hops' well-known role, flavouring beer. The name comes from the Anglo-Saxon *hoppan*, to climb, and hops make a very attractive climber in the garden. A golden variety is particularly interesting, trailing round a tree or arch.

Hops have been used since antiquity, not only for flavouring but for their medicinal properties. The Jewish captives in Babylon drank barley beer flavoured with hops to protect themselves from leprosy, but hops were not used in British breweries till 1524. Henry VIII forbade their use as he said they caused melancholy, and today, hops are best avoided by those who suffer from depressive illnesses. Like opium, they used to be smoked for their narcotic properties. Today the relaxant and sedative effects of hops can be employed internally to ease muscle tension and relieve anxiety, to soothe pain and induce restful sleep. Their relaxant effect is particularly felt in the digestive tract, easing stress-related problems such as spasm and colic as well as nervous indigestion, irritable bowel syndrome and diverticulitis.

How to Grow: Propagate by sowing seeds in late summer or autumn in a cold frame to overwinter. Germination can be erratic. Alternatively, hops can be grown from summer cuttings or divisions of the plant in spring. Prefer rich moist soil in full sun or light shade. Need support. Water freely in dry weather. Can reach 6m (20ft) high and flower July to August, producing fruit September to October.

Hypericum perforatum

St John's Wort

Part used: Leaves and flowers
Contains: Glycosides, flavonoids, tannins, resin, volatile oil

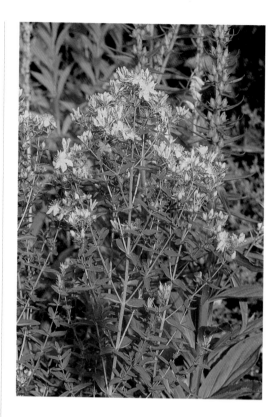

St John's wort is a perennial plant with bright yellow flowers that bloom in midsummer, on or around St John's day. It can be found growing wild in woods and shady places and chalky grassland. The flowers are covered in little black dots which contain a red pigment. If these are soaked in olive oil in a jar on a sunny windowsill, they produce a lovely pinky-red oil, called in the past 'heart of Jesus oil'.

St John's wort's generic name comes from the Greek *huper eikon*, meaning, among other things, 'against an apparition', as the plant was considered effective against the powers of evil and darkness. According to the theory of the Doctrine of Signatures which was expounded by Paracelsus in the sixteenth century, the red juice from the flowers and the tiny perforations in the leaves indicate the plant's efficacy in healing wounds and stemming bleeding. The ancient Greeks and Romans, as well as the Crusaders, took St John's wort into battle with them to staunch bleeding and heal wounds and burns.

St John's wort is still valued for its wonderful healing properties. Used externally, it soothes and heals burns, cuts, wounds, sores and ulcers, as well as sprains, varicose veins, bruises and sunburn. It has an affinity for the nervous system, and when taken internally it eases tension and anxiety and dispels depression. It increases sensitivity to sunlight and has been used for those suffering from seasonal affective disorder (SAD) and jet lag. It is excellent for emotional problems during the menopause and, when used internally and externally, for all kinds of nerve pain. Its antibacterial and antiviral actions make it a useful remedy for a wide range of infections and are currently being investigated for their benefits in treatment of HIV.

NB: Can cause photo-sensitivity in some people.

How to Grow: Propagate by sowing seeds or dividing roots in spring, or taking cuttings in summer. Prefers well-drained soil in either sun or shade. Grows up to 90cm (3ft) high and flowers from mid-to late summer.

Hyssopus officinalis

HYSSOP

Part used: Flowers and leaves
Contains: Volatile oil, resin, gums, silica, bitters, tannins, flavonoid glycosides, sulphur

Hyssop is a hardy evergreen perennial with pretty flowers in either pink, blue, purple or white which are loved by bees. Hyssop makes an excellent low hedging plant and a good companion in the vegetable garden as it attracts cabbage white butterflies away from brassicas and other leafy crops. It can be found growing wild on dry chalky soil.

Hyssop was brought from its native Europe to Britain by Gerard in 1597 and was popular as an edging plant in Tudor knot gardens and mazes. It is mentioned in the Old Testament as a symbol of purity and forgiveness – David said, 'Purge me with hyssop and I shall be clean.' Similarly the ancient Greeks had used it as a holy herb for cleansing ceremonies. The Romans considered it an effective protection against the plague, and in the Middle Ages it was a valuable strewing herb and was used to cleanse houses of sick people.

Today, hyssop is valued for its antimicrobial properties, and when taken internally it can help the immune system's fight against infection, particularly in the respiratory tract. It can be taken hot for colds and flu, to clear catarrh and phlegm in the chest, as well as for chest infections, pleurisy and asthma. It has expectorant and decongestant properties, and by stimulating the circulation it causes sweating, enhancing the elimination of toxins through the pores and bringing down fevers. It makes a good digestive and relaxes the spasms of the gut that cause colic and constipation. It also acts as a tonic to the nervous system, making an excellent restorative.

How to Grow: Propagate by sowing seeds in spring or dividing the plant in spring or autumn, or by taking stem cuttings in summer or autumn. Prefers light, well-drained soil and full sun. Grows up to 60cm (2ft) high and flowers in late summer.

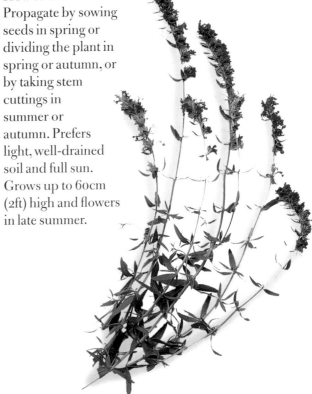

Inula helenium

ELECAMPANE

Part used: Root and rhizome
Contains: Volatile oils, inulin, sterols, resin, pectin, mucilage

Elecampane is a large, handsome perennial plant with large yellow daisy-like flowers and downy leaves that can grow up to 5cm (2in) long. Its bitter and aromatic root was popular for flavouring digestive liqueurs and vermouths, and candied it was used in confectionery.

Elecampane's Latin name comes from Helen of Troy as the plant was said to spring from her tears as they fell to the ground when she was taken away by Paris. It has been valued as a medicine since the time of Hippocrates for digestive problems, asthma, coughs and catarrhal congestion. Galen recommended it for sciatica and Culpeper said it is 'very effectual to warm a cold, windy stomach'.

Today the pungent root of elecampane is used internally as a warming expectorant, excellent for catarrh, colds, asthma, bronchitis and other chest infections. It has antibacterial and antifungal properties and taken hot it helps to bring down fevers and increases the circulation. It has long been popular as a remedy for tuberculosis. Elecampane warms and invigorates the digestion and its bitters stimulate the flow of bile from the liver. It has also been used to expel worms. Used externally elecampane makes a good antiseptic wash for cuts and wounds, and for skin infections such as scabies and herpes.

How to Grow: Propagate by sowing seeds, barely covering them or dividing the roots in spring or autumn. Will grow happily in moist soil and sun or semi-shade. Grows 0.6-1.5m (2-5ft) high and flowers July and August. Makes a good plant for the herb garden or back of flower border. Self-seeds easily if flower heads are left.

Jasminum grandiflorum/Jasminum officinalis

JASMINE

Part used: Flowers
Contains: Resin, salicylic acid, alkaloid, essential oil

The deliciously perfumed jasmine is a perennial climber with pretty star-shaped flowers which have been woven into bridal wreaths, worn in the hair or round the wrists and neck as scented ornaments and used as religious offerings in India for centuries. The oil pressed from the flowers is highly popular in perfumes and hair oils. The common white jasmine, *J. officinalis*, was introduced into Europe in the mid-16th century from India and Persia, while the Spanish jasmine, *J. grandiflorum*, a native of the North Himalayas, is similar with larger, more perfumed flowers.

For centuries in Ayurvedic medicine jasmine has been used for calming the nerves and relieving pain such as in headaches and period pain, as well as for helping the emotional problems that contribute to it. In Malaysia jasmine has long been recommended for uterine infections after childbirth, for fevers and as a nerve sedative. In England Culpeper praised it as a herb to facilitate childbirth, to remedy uterine

ELECAMPANE (*Inula helenium*)

74

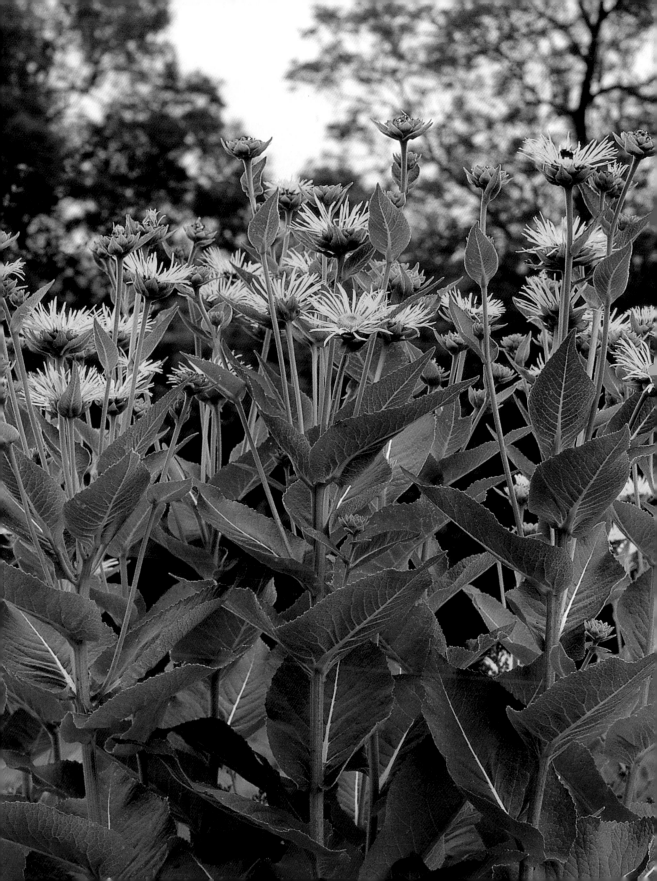

problems and for 'cold and catarrhous conditions'.

Jasmine has an affinity for the female reproductive system and makes a good internal antiseptic remedy for genito-urinary infections including cystitis and salpingitis. Its astringent properties help to reduce heavy bleeding and congestion in the pelvis contributing to period pain. Its calming and relaxant properties help to reduce stress and stress-related problems such as headaches, pre-menstrual syndrome, period pain, and colic, and are excellent during childbirth to soothe pain and ease contractions. In India jasmine is used for cleansing the lymphatic system and, along with other treatments, for Hodgkin's disease and lymphatic cancer. It has a decongestant action in the respiratory system, clearing colds, catarrh and bronchial congestion.

How to Grow: Propagate by taking cuttings in late summer or autumn. Prefers full sun and well-drained fertile soil. Grows 3-5m (10-16ft) and flowers from June to October. Requires support. Prune in autumn after flowering.

Laurus nobilis
SWEET BAY

Part used: Leaves, berries, oil
Contains: Leaves – volatile oil, tannic acid, bitters; Berries – fat, volatile oil

Sweet bay can be grown as an evergreen tree or bush and is much loved for its aromatic leathery leaves, which are a vital ingredient of bouquet garni, and as a decorative shrub in the garden.

The bay tree, or European laurel, was well known and highly respected in the ancient cultures of Greece and Rome. It was dedicated to the god Apollo and the leaves were woven into crowns and presented as symbols of wisdom and victory – today, Britain has a poet laureate as its most eminent poet, while the French examination, the *baccalaureat*, comes from the Latin for laurel berry, *bacca laurens*.

The volatile oils in bay are antiseptic and together with the digestive bitters make this a good internal remedy for stimulating a poor appetite and relieving indigestion, wind and gastro-intestinal infections. The plant has a stimulating effect on the circulation and the dilute oil applied externally makes a good warming rub for arthritis and rheumatic pain. Bay has a warming and expectorant action in the respiratory system, useful for clearing bronchial catarrh and relieving coughs and chest infections.

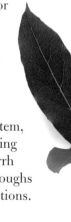

How to Grow: Propagate by taking cuttings in early summer or layering established shrubs in late summer/early autumn. Prefers a sunny, sheltered frost-free site and rich soil. Needs protection in cold winters. Can grow up to 15m (50ft) and produces flowers in late spring or early summer.

Lavendula officinalis

LAVENDER

Part used: Flowers
Contains: Volatile oil, tannins, coumarins, flavonoids, triterpenoids

Fragrant lavender is a much-loved traditional cottage-garden herb, with its evergreen grey-green foliage and spires of highly scented mauve-blue flowers. It is a perennial shrub from the Mediterranean coast, now cultivated in many parts of the world for its popular use in perfumery and aromatherapy. Lavender water is one of the oldest perfumes. It is mentioned in the 12th-century writings of Hildegarde of Bingen, but many centuries earlier the Romans were using lavender to perfume their baths – hence its name, *lavendula*, which comes from *lavare*, 'to wash'.

During the Middle Ages and the Renaissance, lavender was very popular as a strewing herb to perfume and sanitise the floors of houses and churches and to ward off the plague. It was hung in rooms to keep away germ-carrying flies and mosquitoes, much as it was hung in linen cupboards by our grandmothers to scent the clothes and deter moths. Gerard used lavender's medicinal benefits for treating migraine, faintness and 'the panting and passion of the heart', while Mattioli, the 16th-century Italian herbalist, recommended it for 'disorders of the brain due to coldness, such as epilepsy, apoplexy, spasms and paralysis'. Lavender makes a wonderful relaxing remedy for mind and body. Used externally, it calms anxiety and nervousness and relieves stress-related symptoms such as muscle tension, headaches, migraines, palpitations and insomnia. It lifts the spirits and dispels depression and restores strength to those feeling run down. Taken internally, it releases spasm and colic and relieves wind, nausea and indigestion as well as stress-related stomach and bowel problems. Lavender's antibacterial properties help fight off infections such as sore throats, colds, flu and chest infections, while its decongestant action helps to clear phlegm. Taken hot, lavender tea relieves fevers and has a detoxifying effect, increasing elimination of toxins through the skin. Externally, lavender is an excellent antiseptic healer, stimulating tissue repair and minimising scar formation. Lavender oil can be applied neat to burns and scalds, sores and ulcers, and for skin problems such as acne. It also makes a good insect repellent.

How to Grow: Propagate by taking stem cuttings in spring or summer or by dividing the plant in autumn. Alternatively, layer older plants by mounding up soil around the stems. Prefers poor, light, well-drained soil and full sun. Grows up to 90cm (3ft) high and flowers in midsummer. Lavender makes a good low hedging shrub as well as a lovely border plant. Prune in spring or autumn to prevent straggly growth and bare stem.

Leonurus cardiaca

MOTHERWORT

Part used: Leaves and flowers
Contains: Alkaloids, bitter glycosides, tannins, resins, vitamin A

Motherwort is an interesting perennial member of the Labiatae family with its five-lobed leaves and whorls of pinkish flowers. It can be found wild in many parts of Europe, on banks and in hedgerows in gravelly or calcareous soil. It was called *leonurus* since it was thought that the leafy stem resembled a lion's tail.

Motherwort has been praised since the days of the early Greeks as a relaxing remedy for expectant mothers, which accounts for its common name. As a remedy for the womb, it has been prescribed over the centuries for painful or delayed periods and to prepare for childbirth.

It also has an affinity for the heart, hence its Latin name, *cardiaca*, and was considered excellent for strengthening and gladdening the heart and as Culpeper said 'to drive melancholy vapours from the heart.'

Today, motherwort is still recommended to be taken internally for its relaxing and toning effect on the uterus, useful for relieving period pain and regulating periods as well as for preparing for childbirth. It has a mildly sedative effect, good for tension or anxiety about the coming birth, as well as for calming stress-related symptoms such as palpitations and irregular heart rates, and is particularly useful during the menopause. It is a beneficial remedy for the heart and has the ability to lower blood pressure.

NB: Avoid in early pregnancy. Use a few weeks prior to the birth.

How to Grow: Propagate by sowing seeds in spring or autumn, or by dividing roots. Grows 0.9-1.5m (3-5ft) high and flowers midsummer to mid-autumn. Prefers well-drained, light, calcareous soil and full sun. Self-seeds easily.

Related plant
L. sibiricus: Chinese motherwort – a bitter diuretic, simulates uterus and circulation

Levisticum officinalis
LOVAGE

Part used: Dried root, fresh/dried leaves and flowers, seeds
Contains: Essential oil, resin, starch, sugars, tannin, gum, vitamin C, coumarin

Lovage is a handsome, highly aromatic, giant-size perennial, with glossy leaves and umbels of yellowy-green flowers. It has an unusual, pungent flavour; a few leaves can enhance salads, soups and casseroles, while the stems can be cooked like celery or candied like angelica. The seeds can be baked on bread and biscuits and the cooked roots are delicious as a vegetable.

Lovage was popular with the ancient Greeks who chewed the seeds to sweeten their breath, promote appetite and digestion, and relieve wind. The medieval Benedictine monks grew it in monastery gardens for its culinary and medicinal benefits. It was used as a diuretic, for arthritis and rheumatism and to clear catarrh. It was reputed by some to help those in love and was used in love potions and as an aphrodisiac.

The leaves make a deliciously fragrant tea, which promotes the circulation, aids the digestion, brings down fevers and clears catarrh. It has a diuretic action and so acts as a detoxifying remedy, hastening the elimination of toxins from the system via the kidneys.

N.B: Avoid during pregnancy or if suffering from kidney disease.

How to Grow: Propagate by sowing seeds in spring or summer in deep, moist fertile soil, in full sun or light shade. Prefers clay.

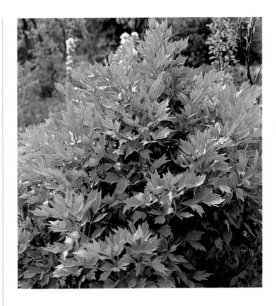

Alternatively, divide the plant in spring or autumn. For a continuous supply of leaves cut back once or twice through the summer. It grows up to 2.4m (8ft) high and flowers June to August.

Related plants
L. Chinensis – root used in Chinese medicine for digestive and menstrual problems

Linum usitatissimum
FLAX/LINSEED

Part used: Oil and seeds
Contains: Fixed oil including linoleic and linolenic acid, mucilage, protein, cyanogenic glycoside

Flax is a slender annual with beautiful blue (sometimes white) flowers, often to be seen in fields resembling stretches of pure blue water, where it is grown for oil and textile production. It is the oldest known cultivated

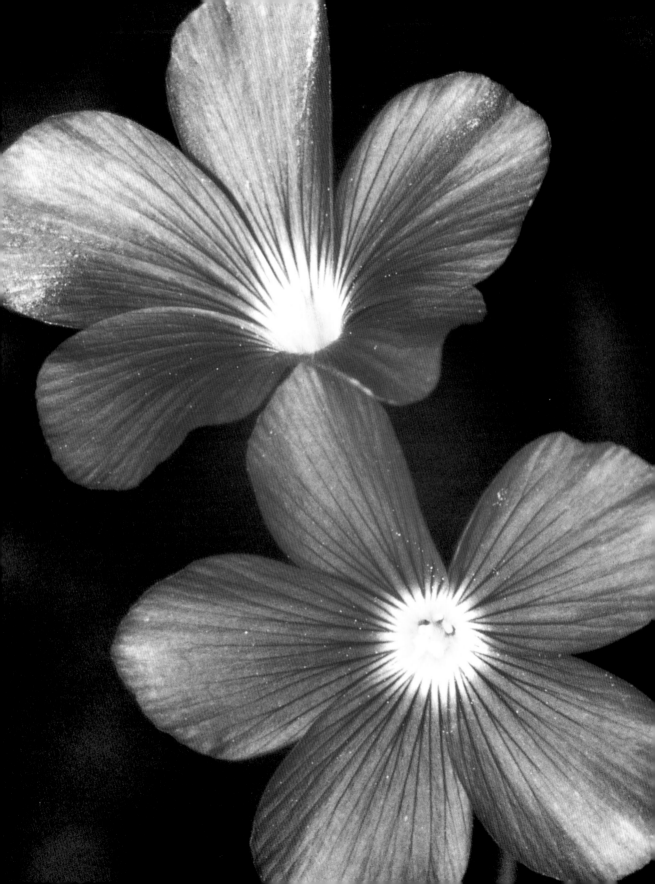

plant, grown for its fibrous stem which was, and still is, used for making linen. Remnants of linen have been found in burial sites dating back to the 23rd century BC.

Flax or linseed has been used as a medicine for thousands of years. Hippocrates used it to soothe irritation and inflammation throughout the body. Linseed tea has long been used for soothing sore throats and troublesome coughs, and poultices of crushed seed were applied externally to draw away inflammation in bronchitis, pneumonia, pleurisy, neuralgia and muscle and joint pain.

Flax seeds are high in oil and mucilage, which, taken internally, soothes mucous membranes and protects them from irritation. In the respiratory system linseed soothes harsh irritating coughs and sore throats; in the digestive system it relieves gastritis, enteritis and colitis. The seeds soaked in water overnight act as an excellent bulk laxative. In the urinary system flax soothes cystitis and irritable bladder. Recently food-grade flax oil has been recommended for drawing heavy metals such as aluminium from the body. Linoleic and linolenic acids are fundamental to the health of skin, blood and kidneys and to the formation of cell membranes and the production of white blood cells and hormones in the body. They also lower blood cholesterol and blood pressure and prevent thrombosis.

How to Grow: Propagate by sowing seeds in late spring or early summer in well-drained or dry soil and full sun. Grows 90cm (3ft) and bears flowers in midsummer followed by pods of oval brown seeds.

FLAX/LINSEED (*Linum usitatissimum*)

Lonicera periclymenum
WILD HONEYSUCKLE

Part used: Leaves and flowers
Contains: Mucilage, glucoside, salicylic acid, invertin

Wild honeysuckle is a woody, deciduous twining shrub or climber, loved by many for its honey-sweet scent that pervades the evening air where it grows. Through the centuries it has inspired many a poet and writer, and its climbing, twining nature has been seen as a symbol of the bonds of affection and being united in love.

'Honeysuckle' is a very old flower name, which goes back to the early 8th century. A syrup of the flowers is an old remedy for asthma, croup and irritating coughs. Gerard recommended it for hardness of the spleen, shortness of breath, hiccoughs and 'wearisomeness'. Culpeper's list of ills remedied by honeysuckle included cramps, convulsions, 'palsies', asthma, 'evil of the spleen' and sunburn. He recommended it for speedy delivery in childbirth.

Today honeysuckle is still valued as a remedy for respiratory infections – taken internally it has anti-inflammatory, expectorant, antibiotic and antispasmodic properties, useful for dealing with spasm and phlegm in the chest as in asthma, croup, whooping cough and bronchitis. The salicylic acid in the plant means that honeysuckle has an aspirin-like action, relieving aches and pains, headaches, flu, fevers, arthritis and rheumatism. Honeysuckle is also a gentle laxative and diuretic, is calming to the nervous system, is good for many stress-related conditions and makes an excellent detoxifying remedy.

NB: Berries are poisonous.

How to Grow: Propagate by sowing seeds in pots in autumn. Germination can be slow. Alternatively you can take cuttings in summer. Prune and mulch with plenty of compost in springtime. Grows in most good soils, in sun or shade. Needs training up walls, trellis, etc. Grows up to 6m (20ft) high and flowers in summer.

Related plants
L. caprifolium – yellow flowers and orange berries, similarly antiseptic, diuretic and expectorant
L. Japonica – vigorous, semi-evergreen climber used widely in Chinese herbal medicine
L. nigra – hardwood shrub, black berries and orange flowers, used in homeopathic medicine

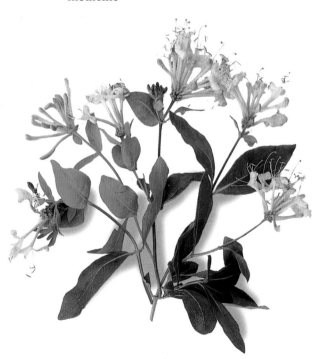

Melissa officinalis
LEMON BALM

Part used: Leaves and flowers
Contains: Volatile oils, polyphenols, tannins, flavonoids, triterpenoids

Lemon balm is a lovely lemon-scented perennial much loved in cottage gardens, particularly for its refreshing taste and smell. The leaves can be added to flavour summer drinks and fruit cups, salads, meat and vegetable dishes, and they make a delicious tea. Lemon balm is loved by bees – *melissa* is Greek for 'bee' – and when planted by beehives it will attract new members to the colony.

Lemon balm was brought to Britain by the Romans where it was a valuable strewing herb and a favourite in the kitchen. It was praised as a wonderful medicine to clear the mind, improve memory and lift the spirits and recommended to Oxford students in the 16th century to drive away 'heaviness of mind' and sharpen the understanding. In the Middle Ages, it was favoured by Arabs in their elixirs of life and in 17th-century Paris, Carmelite nuns made it into Carmelite tea to promote longevity.

Today, lemon balm has proved its benefit to the nervous system and is used internally to lift depression and calm anxiety, release tension and enhance relaxation and restful sleep. It is excellent for improving concentration when studying or working, for soothing stress or exam nerves and relieving nervous headaches and neuralgia. Taken internally, it has a particular affinity for the digestive system, calming tension and soothing irritation and inflammation, and is good for nervous indigestion, colic, wind, nausea, diarrhoea and any stress-related digestive disorder. It calms the heart and relaxes spasm in the reproductive system that causes period pain. Lemon balm can relieve symptoms of PMS and if taken prior to childbirth will ease the birth and lessen pain. In hot tea it reduces fever and clears catarrhal congestion and it is an excellent remedy for a whole range of allergies such as hay fever and eczema.

How to Grow: Propagate by sowing seeds in moist fertile soil and full sun or light shade, or divide the plant in the autumn. Cut back in the summer to encourage a fresh supply of leaves. Grows in clumps up to 90cm (3ft) high and flowers in midsummer. Self-seeds easily. The variegated plant (M. o. var. variegata) is delightful.

Mentha piperita
PEPPERMINT

Part used: Flowers
Contains: Volatile oils, flavonoids, phytol, tocopherols, carotenoids, betaine, azulenes, rosmarianic acid, tannin

Mint is a very popular perennial herb. Today, we know peppermint and spearmint (*M. spicata*) in sweets, chewing gum, tea, toothpaste, mint sauce, mint jelly, cosmetics and, of course, in medicines. There are many different mints, all with similar benefits but generally milder than peppermint in taste, smell and medicinal action.

The use of peppermint in medicine goes back at least 2000 years. Its refreshing taste and smell have been enjoyed all over the world since the time of the ancient Egyptians. Remains of mint have been found in tombs dating back to 3000 BC and the ancient Chinese, Japanese, Egyptians, Greeks and Romans are all recorded as growing it. The name 'mint' comes from the Latin *mente*, meaning 'thought' as garlands of mint were worn in early times to stimulate the brain, concentrate the mind and inspire clear thoughts. The Jews used mint for strewing in synagogues to cleanse and perfume the air for worship. Later Gerard said, 'The smell rejoiceth the heart of man' and 'doth stir up the minde and the taste to a greedy desire for meat.' It was obviously known for its appetite-enhancing properties.

Today, mint makes an excellent digestive remedy, stimulating the appetite and improving digestion and absorption when taken internally. It has a relaxant and anti-inflammatory effect, relieving pain and spasm in the gut, stomach aches, colic, wind, heartburn, indigestion, nausea, vomiting and travel sickness. The tannins protect the digestive tract from irritation and infection and mint is excellent for many bowel disorders such as diarrhoea, Crohn's disease and ulcerative colitis. Taken hot, peppermint tea stimulates the circulation and increases sweating, reducing fevers and clearing catarrhal congestion. Its antiseptic properties help to throw off colds and flu, as well as herpes and chest infections, and its stimulating properties dispel lethargy and help to recharge vital energy.

How to Grow: Propagate by dividing roots in autumn or spring and plant in moist, fertile soil with plenty of potash. Cut back in summer to stimulate growth. Best contained in a pot sunk into the ground to prevent rampant spreading of underground runners. Grows up to 90cm (3ft) and flowers in midsummer. Likes sun or light shade.

Nepeta cataria

CATMINT/CATNIP

Part used: Flowering tops
Contains: Volatile oils, tannins, bitters

Catmint is a hardy perennial with pungent aromatic leaves loved by cats, who roll on it, chew it, even tear it to pieces, hence its name. It is said that if it is grown from seed it is less likely to be damaged by cats than if it is transplanted to the garden as a plant. Catmint grows wild in open places and hedgerows on gravelly or chalky soils. In the garden it makes a good companion plant, deterring harmful insects and beetles, and is loved by bees.

Catmint has been used medicinally at least since Roman times. Pliny said that since snakes hated the smell of catmint, people afraid of snakes should sleep with some by them. The 17th-century herbalists, including Culpeper, recommended catmint for women, for barrenness, to bring on periods and hasten childbirth. Parkinson saw it as a good remedy for bruises and falls.

Today catmint makes an excellent internal

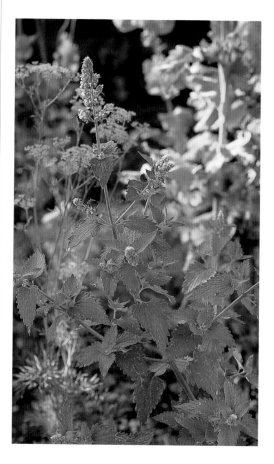

remedy to relax muscle tension. In the uterus it relieves painful periods and reduces stress prior to a period. In the digestive tract it is excellent, particularly for babies with wind or colic. It soothes upset stomachs, indigestion and stress-related problems. Because of its tannins, it is good for diarrhoea and inflammatory bowel problems. In the respiratory system it is helpful for coughs, bronchitis and asthma. It acts as a decongestant and expectorant, and by stimulating circulation it increases perspiration and is good for reducing fevers and bringing out rashes in eruptive infections such as measles and chicken pox.

Externally, it is antiseptic, staunches bleeding and speeds healing of cuts and bites, burns and scalds and bruises.

How to Grow: Propagate by sowing seeds in spring, taking softwood cuttings in spring or dividing the plant in late summer. Prefers well-drained soil and full sun. Grows up to 90cm (3ft) high and flowers June to September. Protect from cats if necessary.

Ocimum basilicum

BASIL

Part used: Leaves
Contains: Essential oil, tannins, basil camphor

Basil is a tender annual with a lovely pungent clove-like fragrance, a favourite in Mediterranean cuisine. It can be grown in pots on a sunny windowsill or in the garden in summer, once all danger of frost has passed, and is delicious, particularly in partnership with tomatoes, in salads, soups, pasta sauces and casseroles. It has been grown in the Mediterranean for thousands of years but was introduced into England only in 1573.

Basil has long been held sacred in India, dedicated to Vishnu, and in ancient Egypt and Greece it was traditionally associated with death, with the power of opening the gates of heaven. The Greeks have for centuries associated basil with courage, carrying it with them on journeys for safety, and with love. It was also used for its

tranquillising properties and to calm the digestion. Later, basil was prepared as snuff to relieve headaches, and Culpeper recommended it for people who had been bitten by 'venomous beasts'.

Taken internally, basil is an excellent relaxing tonic for the nervous system, relieving tension and anxiety and lifting the spirits. It clears the mind and improves concentration and memory, and makes a good remedy for stress-related symptoms such as headaches, nerve pain, indigestion and muscle tension. Taken hot, basil tea acts as a decongestant, well worth taking for colds, flu, catarrh, catarrhal coughs and sore throats. Its antiseptic properties help fight off infections. It has a relaxing effect in the digestive tract, relieving cramp, nausea and constipation, and in the respiratory tract, useful in asthma and tight coughs. Externally, basil leaves can be rubbed on minor cuts, grazes, bites and stings.

How to Grow: Propagate by sowing seeds under glass or indoors in spring; transplant to garden or outside pots once all danger of frosts is past. Prefers rich damp soil and full sun, in a sheltered position. Grows up to 60cm (2ft) high and flowers in mid-to late summer. Removing flowers as they appear will stimulate bushy leaf growth.

Oenothera biennis

EVENING PRIMROSE

Part used: Stems, leaves, seeds and oil
Contains: Whole plant – tannins, mucilage, resin, bitters, potassium. Seeds – essential fatty acids, notably gamma linoleic acid (GLA)

Evening primrose is a handsome biennial plant with sweetly scented cup-shaped pale-yellow flowers that generally open at dusk to attract pollinating insects and night-flying moths. The plant was originally brought to Britain in 1614 from North and South America, via the botanic gardens in Padua, for its culinary virtues. The fresh young leaves were eaten in salads and the seeds were used for food and oil. The fleshy root of the first year's growth can be boiled like a vegetable and tastes nutty, a bit like parsnip.

Evening primrose was familiar to the ancient Greeks, and Theophrastus (350 BC) gave its generic name, from *oinos*, 'wine', and *thera*, 'hunt', as the plant was said either to stimulate a taste for wine or to have the power to neutralise the effects of drinking too much of it. The North American Indians used it externally to apply to bruises and cuts, and took it internally for obesity.

The stems and leaves are rich in mucilage which is soothing when used externally for skin eruptions and internally for irritated conditions of the digestive tract. Their mild sedative effect helps to relieve nervous tension. It is the oil from the seeds, however, that has excited so much attention and provoked such extensive research in the last 15 to 20 years. Taken internally, the fatty acids are vital for a healthy immune system and normal hormonal function, and very helpful in treatment of allergies such as eczema, hyperactivity, asthma and migraine, as well as PMS and menopausal problems. They encourage regeneration of a damaged liver and help to counteract the effects of excess alcohol, as well as withdrawal symptoms in alcoholics. Evening primrose oil has also been shown to be beneficial when treating arthritis, high blood pressure and raised cholesterol.

How to Grow:
Propagate by sowing seeds in summer in well-drained soil and full sun. Self-seeds easily. First year, it produces a rosette of bright green leaves and in the second year it grows up to 1.2m (4ft) high and flowers from midsummer to mid-autumn.

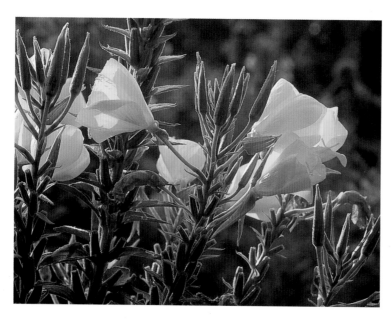

Origanum marjorana
SWEET MARJORAM

Part used: Flowers and leaves
Contains: Essential oil, mucilage, bitters, tannins, antioxidants

Sweet marjoram is the most sweetly scented of all the marjorams, and the most handsome with its white flowers and grey-green leaves. It is a half-hardy annual in cool temperate areas and a perennial in warmer areas of Europe and America, growing wild in sunny places. All marjorams are highly aromatic and very popular in the kitchen as well for decorating the garden.

Marjoram is a very ancient medicine, loved by the Greeks – in fact its botanical name comes from the Greek *oras* for 'mountain' and *ganos* for 'joy'. They used it to nourish the brain and remedy the digestion, and in cases of narcotic poisoning, convulsions and dropsy. Gerard said that marjoram 'cureth them that have drunk opium'. In medieval monasteries the monks grew marjoram as an anaphrodisiac, to help prevent sexual desire. It was a popular strewing herb in Tudor times, for warding off disease and infestation.

Today, marjoram makes a good internal warming and relaxing remedy, to improve the circulation and relieve anxiety, nervousness, insomnia and depression, as well as stress-related symptoms such as headaches, abdominal pain, indigestion, PMS, period pain and muscular pain. As a diuretic it relieves fluid retention and hastens elimination of wastes from the body, which makes it a good remedy for arthritis and gout. Its antimicrobial properties help to fight off infections such as colds, sore throats, flu, chest infections and herpes simplex. Taken hot, it reduces fevers and acts as an effective decongestant. The antioxidants help to protect the body from the impact of the ageing process.

How to Grow: Propagate by sowing seeds under glass and plant out in late spring once all danger of frost has passed. Alternatively, take stem cuttings in summer or divide the root in autumn and overwinter in a frost-free area. Prefers light well-drained soil and full sun. Grows up to 25cm (10in) high and flowers in late summer to early autumn.

Passiflora incarnata
PASSIONFLOWER

Part used: Vine and flower
Contains: Alkaloids, sugar, gum, sterols, flavonoids, coumarin derivatives, essential oil

Passionflower is a fast-growing perennial climber with one of the most intricate and interesting flowers in the plant kingdom. It derives its lovely name from the resemblance of the corona in the centre of the flower to the crown of thorns worn by Christ, and of the stamen and pistil formation to the cross. It bears yellowish, edible fruits called maypops, filled with sweet soft flesh and seeds.

Passionflower is indigenous to North America and maypop seeds have been found by archeologists at Native American camp sites over 5000 years old. It was discovered growing in Peru in 1605 by Spanish explorers and missionaries and sent to Pope Paul V because of its religious connotations.

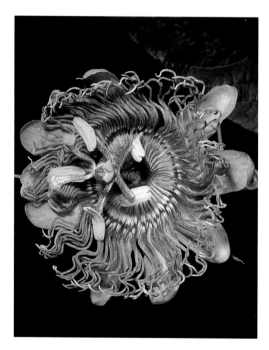

Passionflower is an excellent relaxant and sedative and its internal use should be considered in all stress-related or painful conditions. It will calm nervous anxiety and agitation and soothe pain including headaches, neuralgia, shingles, muscular aches and period pains. It is one of the best herbal tranquillisers for chronic insomnia and is completely non-addictive. It can also be used for Parkinson's disease, muscle twitching and cramps, high blood pressure and colic. Its relaxing effects in the chest relieve irritating and nervous coughs, croup and asthma.

How to Grow: Propagate by sowing seeds in spring, by layering, by taking cuttings in September, or by dividing runners in autumn. It thrives in relatively poor, sandy, slightly acidic soils and needs good drainage, full sun and a place to climb. Can reach 10m (30ft) high and flowers through the summer and bears fruit in early autumn.

Petroselinum crispum

PARSLEY

Part used: Leaves, root, seeds
Contains: Essential oil, flavonoids, glycoside, vitamins and minerals

Parsley, the most popular of culinary herbs, is a hardy biennial, often grown as an annual. The familiar-tasting leaves are highly nutritious, rich in vitamins A, B and C and in minerals including iron, calcium, magnesium, manganese and sodium, as well as essential fatty acids.

Parsley was also popular among the ancient Greeks and Romans and was dedicated to Persephone, Queen of the Underworld.

It was eaten at funeral banquets and planted on graves to bring good luck to the departed. The Romans carried parsley for protection and gave it to gladiators to eat before a fight to promote strength, cunning and agility. In early European herbal traditions parsley was well known as a remedy for liver problems, jaundice, fluid retention, urinary stones and malaria.

Taken internally, parsley stimulates the appetite and improves digestion and absorption and makes a good nutritious tonic when feeling run down and for anaemia. Its relaxing effect relieves colic, wind and nervous indigestion as well as headaches, migraine, asthma and irritable bladder. Its antiseptic volatile oils, notably apiol, help combat infections. Parsley stimulates the kidneys and acts as a diuretic, useful in urinary infections and fluid retention, and for clearing the toxins from the body that contribute to arthritis and gout. Parsley stimulates the muscles of the uterus, promoting contractions during childbirth, and increases the supply of breast milk in nursing mothers. It also stimulates the circulation and acts as a tonic to the nervous system, relieving anxiety and depression.

NB: Avoid during pregnancy or if suffering from kidney disease.

How to Grow: To propagate, first soak seeds for 24 hours in warm water and then sow seed under glass or outdoors in late spring. Do not cover with soil. Sow again in midsummer for winter use or for pots indoors. Prefers moist fertile soils and sun or light shade. Grows 75cm (2ft 6in) high and bears flowers in mid-to late summer.

Polygonum bistorta

BISTORT

Part used: Fresh leaves, dried rhizome
Contains: Tannins, vitamin C, starch, oxalic acid

Bistort is an attractive perennial plant with tall spikes of pink flowers. It can be found growing wild in many areas of Europe and North America in damp grassland. It used to be a popular garden plant as the leaves and tender shoots were cooked as a vegetable, particularly in the north of England, where bistort pudding was traditionally eaten at Easter.

Bistort has been valued as a medicine since the Renaissance, when the leaves and roots were used to counteract poisons and to treat ague (malaria) and intermittent fevers.

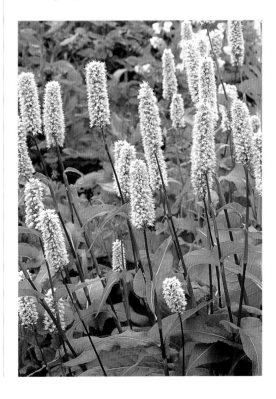

Dried and powdered it was applied to cuts and wounds to staunch bleeding, and a decoction in wine was taken for internal bleeding and diarrhoea. It was also given to cause sweating and drive out the plague, smallpox, measles and other infectious diseases.

Bistort is rich in tannins and is one of the best astringents in the plant kingdom. Taken internally, it is excellent for bleeding, such as from nosebleeds, heavy periods and wounds, and for diarrhoea and dysentery. Since it reduces inflammation and mucous secretions it makes a good remedy for colitis and for catarrhal congestion. Bistort can be used as a gargle for sore throats and a mouthwash for sore, bleeding gums and mouth ulcers. Externally, it is a fine remedy for haemorrhoids, varicose veins and ulcers.

How to Grow: Propagate by sowing seeds or by dividing the roots in autumn or spring and planting out in rich, moisture-retentive soil, in sun or shade. Grows 30-45cm (12-18in) high and flowers in May and June, and often again in September and October. It makes a good ornamental plant in borders, around ponds and in the herb garden, particularly when grown in large clumps.

Primula veris
COWSLIP

Part used: Roots and flowers
Contains: Saponins, salicylates, flavonoids, volatile oil

Cowslips are a beautiful but now rather rare feature of chalky meadows and hedgerows. They are popularly believed to be the favourite flower of the nightingale, which apparently sings only where cowslips flourish. These sweet-smelling perennials have been overpicked in the past when gallons of flowers were gathered for making wines, syrups, conserves, cordials, cheese, puddings and creams.

Cowslip was valued by the old herbalists for remedying paralysis, earning its old name *herba paralysis*. It was also used as a remedy for a whole host of nervous afflictions including vertigo, convulsions, nerve pain, and, according to Culpeper, 'false apparitions'. Parkinson recommended cowslip water to cleanse the skin and clear spots and wrinkles, while others have taken cowslip tea for migraine, insomnia and general debility.

Today, cowslip root and flowers are used internally as a relaxing and sedative remedy for nervous tension, anxiety, insomnia and as a general tonic to the nervous system. They are excellent for stress-related problems such as headaches, muscular aches and pains and nerve pain and have a reputation for lifting the spirits and dispelling depression. Taken hot, cowslips relieve fevers and have a decongestant and expectorant action, good for colds, flu, sore throats, coughs and catarrh. The salicylates in the root have an anti-inflammatory action, useful when treating arthritis and gout.

How to Grow: Propagate from sowing seeds under glass in trays or in a nursery bed, or divide roots in autumn. Prefers chalky soil, but will grow in most soils, and in full sun or semi-shade. Grows up to 12-22cm (5-9in) high and flowers in April and May.

COWSLIP (*Primula veris*)

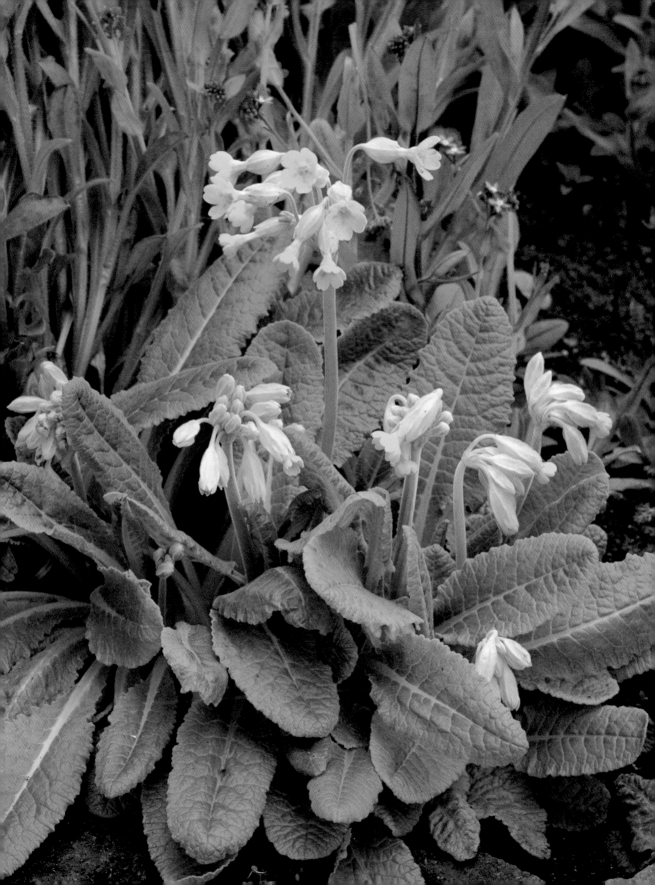

Pulmonaria officinalis

LUNGWORT

Part used: Leaves and flowers
Contains: Mucilage, saponins, allantoin, tannin, silica, potassium, iron and other minerals

Lungwort is a pretty, downy perennial member of the borage family with bell-shaped flowers, first pink and then blue, white or purple, appearing as one of the first flowers in early spring. It can be found growing wild in woods and hedgerows,

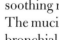

particularly on chalky soil, and is a popular garden plant for ground cover in shady areas. The young leaves can be eaten in soups and stews as well as added to salads.

The hairy green leaves, mottled with silver, were thought to resemble the lungs, and according to the Doctrine of Signatures lungwort has been valued as a remedy for a variety of respiratory problems. In 17th-century England lungwort was known as Jerusalem cowslip and was held in high esteem for treating the spots on the lungs which occur in tuberculosis, as well as for asthma and bronchitis.

Today, lungwort is still used internally as a soothing remedy for harsh irritating coughs. The mucilage soothes irritation of the bronchial tubes and the silica speeds healing. Its expectorant properties help to expel phlegm from the chest, while the astringent tannins reduce catarrhal secretions. Externally, the silica and allantoin have wonderful healing properties, while the tannins stem bleeding, making lungwort a useful remedy for cuts and wounds, burns and scalds, sores and ulcers, varicose veins and haemorrhoids.

How to Grow: Propagate by dividing plants after flowering, in spring or in autumn. Prefers light soils and shade, or semi-shade. It is best lifted and divided every 4 to 5 years. Grows 30cm (1ft) high and flowers in early spring.

Related plants
P. saccharata: Bethlehem sage – a larger plant with similar leaves, often grown for its greeny-silvery foliage; has similar medicinal uses

Rosa sp.

ROSE

Part used: Hips, leaves, flowers
Contains: Tannins, pectin, carotene, fruit acids, fatty oil, nicotinamide, vitamins C, B, E, K.

The beautiful perennial perfumed rose, the symbol of love and beauty, has inspired gardeners, poets and artists for thousands of years. The first historical evidence of growing roses can be traced back to around 2600 BC when the king of the Sumerians apparently brought back a 'tree of roses' from an exhibition. Rose petals have been strewn in rivers and decorated palaces of the Moghul emperors, they have formed soft, aromatic carpets for the feasts and banquets of the Greeks and Romans and have filled Roman fountains and baths. Roses were brought to England by the Romans, who planted red and white roses and scattered rose petals on the graves of their loved ones.

Roses have been praised throughout history, not only for their beauty but also for their medicinal qualities. The Greeks considered roses a tonic, and the Roman scholar Pliny the Elder listed at least 32 different preparations of roses for a variety of ailments including the bites of mad dogs. John Gerard said they had cooling properties and that the distilled water of roses 'mitigateth the paine of the eies proceeding from a hot cause, bringeth sleep', and was also good for strengthening the heart and refreshing the spirit.

Today, rose leaves and petals are still used internally for their cooling properties. Taken as a tea they help to bring down fevers and clear heat and toxins from the body that give rise to skin rashes and other inflammatory problems. Roses act to enhance the efforts of the immune system and the tea will help clear cold and flu symptoms, sore throats, catarrh and chest infections. In the digestive tract they help re-establish the normal bacterial population when it has been disrupted by antibiotics or poor diet. Rose hips, petals and oil have a restoring effect on the nervous system, lifting the spirits and calming anxiety. They have an affinity with the female reproductive system, relieving pelvic congestion and pain and heavy periods, and enhancing sexual desire. They are truly the food of love!

How to Grow: Propagation. This hardy perennial can be grown from cuttings taken in late summer. It prefers well-drained, moderately fertile soil and sun or light shade. Repeat-flowering roses should be deadheaded to stimulate further flower development. Roses can be pruned in either autumn or early spring.

Rosmarinus officinalis
ROSEMARY

Part used: Leaves and flowers
Contains: Volatile oils, flavonoids, phenolic acids, tannins, bitters, resins

Rosemary is an attractive hardy evergreen shrub with delightfully aromatic leaves, found growing wild on dry rocky slopes in the Mediterranean, especially near the sea. It is a popular herb in cottage and herb gardens, as well as in the kitchen, where it is used to flavour chicken, lamb and vegetable dishes. To add interest in the garden there are several different varieties of rosemary including Suffolk blue, Majorcan pink, Miss Jessop's upright, Prostatus and Severn Sea, and all are loved by bees.

Rosemary has been held sacred and valued for its medicinal virtues since at least the time of the ancient Egyptians. As a symbol of remembrance the pharaohs placed rosemary in their tombs, and centuries later Shakespeare's Ophelia said 'Here's rosemary for remembrance.' It was considered excellent for the brain, and to dispelling melancholy, and was worn in a cloth around the arm to make the wearer 'light and merrie'. It was grown in the early physic and apothecaries' gardens. Culpeper recommended it for troublesome coughs, while Gerard prescribed it for stuffiness in the head.

Today, rosemary is highly popular as a tonic to the nervous system, increasing circulation to the brain, heightening concentration and improving memory. It is also taken internally to dispel depression, relieve anxiety and strengthen the nerves, excellent for nervous exam students and interviewees. It is considered one of the best remedies for headaches and migraine. Its antimicrobial properties enhance the immune system's fight against infection, and a hot tea will help relieve colds, flu, catarrh, sore throats and chest infections. Rosemary invigorates the digestion and enhances liver and gall bladder function and helps to detoxify the system through its action on the liver and as a diuretic. The tannins are astringent, checking bleeding, relieving diarrhoea and heavy periods, and protecting mucous membranes throughout the body from irritation and inflammation. Externally, rosemary oil makes a wonderfully relieving rub for arthritis and rheumatism.

How to Grow: Propagate by sowing seeds in spring, or taking tip cuttings during summer and early autumn. Prefers a slightly alkaline, well drained soil, full sun and a sheltered position, as some forms are slightly tender. Grows up to 3m (10ft) high and flowers in April and May.

Rubus idaeus

RASPBERRY

Part used: Leaves, fruit
Contains: Leaves – fragarine, tannin, volatile oil, pectin, minerals and trace elements; fruit – sugars, citric and malic acid, vitamins A, B, C, E, pectin, volatile oil, iron, calcium, phosphorous

The perennial raspberry plant has long been known for its delicious fruit, probably since prehistoric times according to remnants found in Swiss archeological excavations. It can be found growing wild in woodland clearings and hedgerows and has been cultivated since the Middle Ages. *Rubus* is Latin for 'red' and *idaeus* means 'of Mount Ida', where it was found growing prolifically.

Raspberries have long been used in refreshing summer drinks, to reduce fevers and diarrhoea and as gargles for sore throats. Raspberry leaves have been valued for their astringent properties and also used in gargles for sore throats, mouthwashes for inflamed gums and lotions for wounds and ulcers, burns and scalds. They were given to relieve diarrhoea and were best known as a parturient, to prepare women for childbirth.

In the last three months of pregnancy, raspberry leaves can be taken as a tea to help tone the uterine and pelvic muscles and prepare them for childbirth. By relaxing

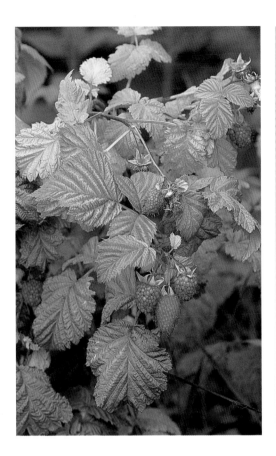

Salvia officinalis
SAGE

Part used: Leaves
Contains: Volatile oils, tannins, phenolic acids, flavonoids, oestrogenic substances

Sage is a popular evergreen perennial shrub, with aromatic soft velvety leaves and whorls of violet-blue flowers. It can be found growing wild on hillsides and grassland in warm regions such as Greece. It is a favourite culinary herb, famous for sage and onion stuffing, and also a much-loved decorative shrub for the garden in its various cultivated forms.

The ancient Greeks knew sage as the immortality herb as it was said to cure so many ills. The Egyptians respected sage as a giver and saver of life and treated plague victims with it. The Romans thought that it enhanced female fertility. In the Middle Ages it was included in many a prescription for longevity and the elixir of life.

Taken internally, sage makes an excellent remedy for infections, with its antibacterial and antifungal properties, and can be taken for colds, flu, fevers, sore throats and chest infections. It was an old remedy for tuberculosis and bronchitis. Its diuretic properties make it a good detoxifying remedy, useful for treating arthritis and gout. In the digestive tract it relaxes tension and colic, stimulates appetite and enhances digestion, and has a beneficial effect on the liver. Sage can be taken for irregular, scanty or painful periods and its oestrogenic properties make it a good remedy for menopausal problems, particularly night sweats and hot flushes. Externally it is an excellent antiseptic first-aid remedy for cuts, wounds, burns, sores, ulcers and sunburn.

over-tense muscles and toning over-relaxed muscles, raspberry leaves enable the uterus to contract effectively during childbirth, easing and speeding the birth. Taken afterwards, they stimulate the flow of breast milk and speed healing of the womb. Raspberries are nutritious and useful in pregnancy to help combat anaemia.

How to Grow: Propagate by planting suckers and taking root cuttings. Canes are best cut down to allow new growth. Prefers moist, rich soil and full sun. Grows 0.9-1.5m (3-5ft) high and flowers in early to midsummer, producing fruit in July. Plant canes 60cm (2ft) apart in rows allowing 1.2-1.5m (4-5ft) between rows.

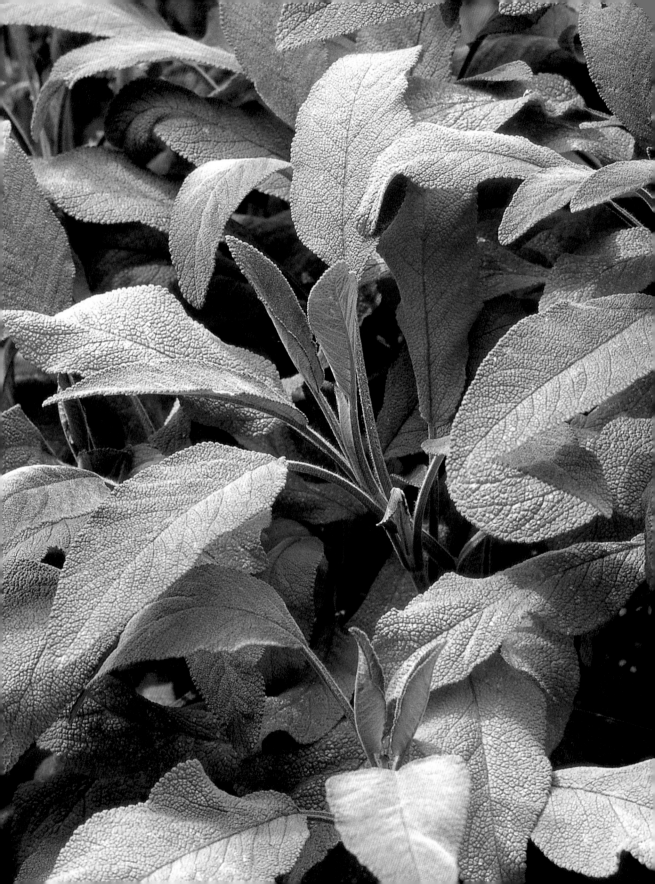

NB: Avoid during pregnancy and while breast feeding.

How to Grow: Propagate by sowing seeds in spring or by taking tip cuttings from spring to autumn, or by layering older bushes. Prefers light, well-drained soil and full sun. Grows up to 75cm (2ft 6in) high and flowers in early summer. To stimulate bushy growth, nip off new shoots. Sage will need renewing every 4 to 5 years as it tends to become rather leggy or woody.

Salvia sclarea

CLARY SAGE

Part used: Leaves and flowers, seeds
Contains: Volatile oil, bitters, tannins, mucilage

Clary sage is an attractive biennial with large velvety leaves and purple-blue flowers, which can be found growing wild on dry chalky pastures. It was used for its wonderful nutty smell and taste by wine merchants in Germany, who added elderflowers and clary sage to ordinary white wine to make it taste like the more expensive muscatel. It was found, however, to induce dangerous levels of intoxication and severe hangovers.

Clary sage has been used medicinally since the days of the ancient Greeks. Its name *clary/sclarea* comes from the Latin *claris,* meaning 'clear', and its old name, 'clear eye', reflects the seed's use for treating irritation and inflammation of the eye and clearing the sight. In Culpeper's day the fresh leaves were enjoyed for their culinary as well as medicinal virtues: 'The fresh

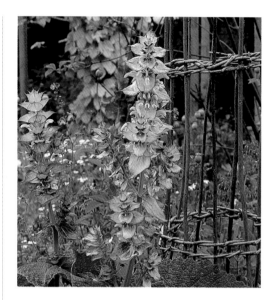

SAGE (*Salvia officinalis Purpurascens*)

leaves dipped in Batter of floure, egs and a littel milk, and fried in Butter and served to the Table, is not unpleasant to any, but exceedingly profitable to those that are troubled with weak backs.'

Today, clary sage makes a good relaxant and tonic to the nerves when taken internally, and internal use is also recommended for stress-related problems such as headaches, insomnia and indigestion. It relieves pain and spasm in the digestive tract and uterus, easing colic, period pains and contractions during childbirth. It has a strengthening action, reducing tiredness and exhaustion and lifting depression, particularly after childbirth. It is beneficial to the chest, for asthma and harsh irritating coughs, and also for excessive perspiration – useful during the menopause especially since it has oestrogenic properties. It makes a soothing lotion for the eyes.

NB: Avoid during pregnancy and do not mix with alcohol.

How to Grow: Propagate by sowing seeds in spring in rich soil and full sun. Grows about 90cm (3ft) high and flowers June to August. Self-seeds easily.

Related plants

S. viridis/horminum – annual similar to clary sage often grown as a bedding plant. Has similar action.

S. praetensis: Meadow sage – similar to clary sage, but less significant. Also useful for eye problems

Sambucus nigra

ELDER

Part used: Flowers, leaves, berries
Contains: Flowers – tannins, flavonoids, essential oil, mucilage, triterpenes; berries – sugar, vitamin C, bioflavonoids, fruit acids; leaves, cyanogenic glycosides, vitamins, tannins, resins, fats, sugars

The fragrant elder tree is gaining in popularity as its delightful elderflower

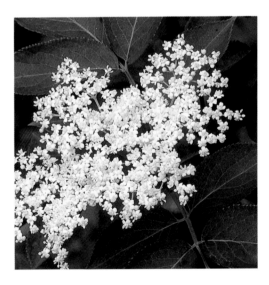

cordial and wine become more widely known. Its abundance of white flowers scent the countryside in early summer, making it an attractive tree for the garden, alone or in hedging . Its ornamental varieties (white, gold, variegated) are very rewarding to grow.

The elder is a legendary tree, considered sacred and magical in folklore and myths and deserving of great respect. It has been called the 'medicine chest of the country people' and was described by the 17th-century diarist John Evelyn as a tree providing a remedy for almost every ill. The flowers were used particularly for fevers and infections as well as for dispelling melancholy and anxiety, while hot elderberry wine on cold winter's nights made a delicious cure for colds.

When hot, elderflower tea is excellent taken internally at the first signs of colds and fevers, sore throats and flu. It increases the circulation and causes sweating, helping to eliminate toxins and bring down fevers. By bringing out the rash in eruptive infections such as measles and chicken pox, it speeds recovery. The decongestant and relaxant effect of elderflowers is helpful in catarrh, as well as in asthma and tight coughs. The flowers' diuretic action, clearing heat and toxins via the urinary system, often helps relieve arthritis and gout. Elderflower tea or distilled elderflower water makes a good external toning lotion for the skin and a remedy for skin problems and sunburn.

How to Grow: Propagate by sowing ripe berries in autumn or taking hardwood cuttings in summer or early autumn. Prefers fertile soil, sun or semi-shade, and grows up to 8m (25ft) high, flowering May and June and producing fruit August to November. Self-seeds easily.

Saponaria officinalis
SOAPWORT

Part used: Root, rhizome and leaves
Contains: Saponins, resin, gum, mucilage, flavonoids, vitamin C

Soapwort is a handsome perennial with large pale-pink flowers, well known in the past as a source of soap. The roots and leaves when boiled in water produce a soapy lather which was used traditionally for washing cloth, particularly in the textile trade. Soapwort can still be used as a natural soap base for home-made soaps and shampoos and is used today for cleaning old and delicate tapestries. The hormone-like saponins lower the surface tension of water, thereby producing a lather.

Soapwort has been used as a medicine for liver complaints, probably since the time of Dioscorides, and as a cleansing remedy for arthritis and rheumatism as well as for skin complaints. It was particularly recommended for 'the itch' related to venereal disease.

Today, soapwort is recommended for use only under professional supervision, as internally, large doses are purgative and mildly poisonous. In small doses it has a laxative and expectorant action, and stimulates the flow of bile from the liver. Its detoxifying properties make it useful in the treatment of gout, arthritis and rheumatism, while the saponins have an anti-inflammatory effect. Soapwort has been used internally and externally for skin conditions such as psoriasis, acne, boils and eczema. In India the prepared root is used to stimulate milk flow in nursing mothers.

How to Grow: Propagate by sowing seeds in early autumn and cover lightly with soil. Germination usually occurs in spring but tends to be erratic. Prefers good fertile soil and full sun, will need support as it grows. Reaches a height of 30-60cm (1-2ft) and flowers from July to September.

Scutellaria laterifolia
VIRGINIAN SKULLCAP

Part used: Leaves and flowers
Contains: Flavonoid glycosides, volatile oil, bitters, tannin, minerals including calcium, potassium and magnesium

Virginian skullcap is a hardy perennial found growing wild in damp places in North America, so named because the calyx of the little blue flower resembles a tiny cap. Common skullcap (*S. galericulata*) and lesser skullcap (*S. minor*) grow wild in

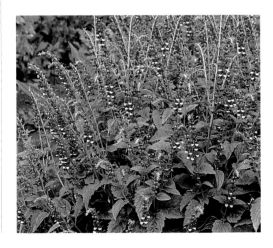

similar sites in Britain and make a pretty addition to a herb garden or border.

Traditionally, the skullcaps have provided effective remedies for a whole range of nervous disorders, including nervousness, agitations, insomnia, hysteria, epilepsy, convulsions and St Vitus dance. Virginian skullcap earned a reputation as a cure for hydrophobia or rabies and in many places was known as mad-dog skullcap. Skullcaps were also used for infertility and to quieten unwanted sexual desires.

Skullcap is rich in nutrients essential to the healthy functioning of the nervous system and taken internally is a perfect tonic for supporting us in our busy, stressful lives. It relaxes and soothes the nerves, and by releasing tension, eases tense, aching muscles. It reduces anxiety and agitation, lifts depression, helps to dispel tiredness and exhaustion and promotes sleep. A great remedy when feeling nervously overwrought or run down and when wanting to stay off or withdraw from orthodox tranquillisers and antidepressants. Good for painful conditions, such as nervous headaches, period pain and arthritis, as well as palpitations, epilepsy, digestive problems and, when taken hot, for fevers.

How to Grow: To propagate sow seeds in moist fertile ground in spring or divide the roots in spring or autumn. Likes a sunny position. *S. galericulata* grows up to 30cm (1ft) and flowers June to September.

Related plants
S. baikalensis Georgi – this plant is found in Siberia, Russia, North China and Japan, is used in Chinese and Tibetan medicine as a stimulant, nerve tonic and sedative.

Silybum/Carduus marianus
MILK THISTLE

Part used: Seeds
Contains: Essential oil, tyramine, histamine, bitters, flavonoids, silymarine

Milk thistle is a very attractive, prickly annual or biennial with glossy green leaves with clear milk-white veins, and red-purple thistle-like flowers. The young shoots and leaves are edible and considered a delicacy by the Arabs. The long tap roots can be cooked like parsnips, the unopened flower heads eaten like artichokes and the seedlings added to salads. It makes a very interesting feature in a herb garden or flower border and is loved by bees and butterflies.

According to medieval legend, the milk-white veins on the leaves of milk thistle come from the milk of the Virgin Mary, and so the plant was dedicated to Mary and called Our Lady's thistle. The diarist John Evelyn

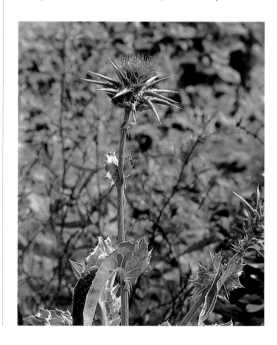

recorded that it was esteemed for its ability to promote breast milk, and Gerard considered it one of the best cures for melancholy. Culpeper recommended milk thistle for preventing and curing the plague, for agues and problems of the liver and spleen, and as a blood-cleansing spring tonic.

For over 2,000 years milk thistle has been valued as a liver remedy, used for jaundice, chronic liver disease and acute hepatitis. This history has stimulated extensive modern research into its amazing liver-protecting properties. It is used internally to treat alcohol-induced cirrhosis, as well as deathcap mushroom poisoning, toxic liver damage and chronic liver disease, including chronic hepatitis and fatty degeneration. It has both preventative and curative properties. It is an excellent digestive and has been used to prevent travel sickness.

How to Grow: Propagate by sowing seeds in spring or autumn in any well-drained soil and full sun. Grows 0.3-1.5m (1-5ft) high and flowers in late summer. Self-seeds easily.

Solidago virgaurea

GOLDENROD

Part used: Flowering tops, leaves
Contains: Saponins, flavonoids, tannins, essential oil

Goldenrod is a familiar herbaceous perennial with its bright yellow, powdery flowers, found growing wild in woods and hedgerows. It is grown as an ornamental in many cultivated forms and is the official state flower of Alabama, Kentucky and Nebraska. All species of goldenrod contain a sap which

Thomas Edison hoped to make into a rubber substitute.

Goldenrod's botanical name comes from the Latin *solidare* meaning 'to make whole' as the plant was used to staunch bleeding and heal wounds and was once called woundwort. In the 16th century, goldenrod was imported from America and sold in London markets until Gerard discovered it growing in Hampstead woods, north of London. The Native Americans used a lotion from the flowers for bee stings and the flowers were added to steam baths to allay pain.

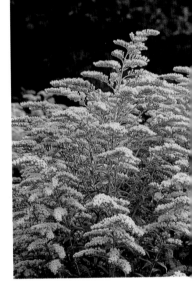

Goldenrod has astringent and diuretic properties and is popular, taken internally, as a remedy for diarrhoea as well as for urinary infections and stones. By hastening elimination of toxins via the urine it will often help relieve arthritis and gout. Taken as a hot tea, it will bring down fevers and help to clear catarrhal congestion as well as relieve colic, nausea and period pains. Externally, a lotion will stem bleeding and speed healing of wounds and ulcers.

How to Grow: Propagate by sowing seeds in autumn or spring, covering only lightly with soil. Alternatively, divide plants in autumn or spring. Prefers light, well-drained soil, full sun or light shade. Spreads rapidly to form clumps. Grows 30-60cm (1-2ft) high and flowers July to September.

Symphytum officinale
COMFREY

Part used: Root
(external use only),
leaves
Contains: Mucilage,
tannins, allantoin,
resin, pyrrolizidine
alkaloids, essential oil,
beta-sitosterol,
triterpenoids, vitamin
B12, protein, zinc

Comfrey is a stout
hairy perennial with
pretty bell-shaped
flowers, found growing in
ditches, streams, and other damp places. It is
a favourite cottage garden herb and is
cultivated in various selected forms for
ornamental gardens. The young leaves and
shoots can be eaten as a vegetable, the wilted
leaves make an excellent mulch for the soil in
garden borders, and the leaves steeped in
water for three to four weeks produce a
nutritious fertiliser, particularly good for
potatoes and tomatoes.

Comfrey has been highly valued for
thousands of years for its wonderful ability
to promote repair of wounds, ulcers and
fractured and broken bones. Its country
names – knit bone, bruisewort and boneset –
reflect its reputation. Culpeper said that
comfrey plants are 'so powerful to
consolidate and knit together that if they be
boiled with dessevered pieces of flesh in a
pot, it will join them together again'!

Comfrey contains a substance, allantoin,
which is a remarkable cell proliferant, known
to stimulate the production of cells
responsible for forming collagen and
connective tissue, cartilage and
bone. So wherever there is damage
or injury to such tissue, comfrey can
speed repair. Used externally, it is the prime
first-aid remedy for healing cuts and
wounds, burns and scalds, sores and
ulcers, with minimal scar formation.

NB: Due to recent controversy
surrounding comfrey root, this is best
avoided for internal use.

How to Grow: Propagate by dividing roots
in early spring or late summer and planting
in moist fertile soil. Root cuttings can also be
taken in spring. Grows up to 0.9-1.8m (3-6ft)
and flowers in purple, blue, pink or white,
through the summer. Comfrey may need
some containing as it can become invasive.

Related plants
S. ×uplandicum: Russian comfrey – has
similar properties

*Tanacetum parthenium/
Pyrethrum
parthenium/Chrysanthemum
parthenium*
FEVERFEW

Part used: Leaves and flowers
Contains: Sesquiterpene lactones, volatile
oils, tannins, bitter resin, pyrethrin

Feverfew is an attractive hardy perennial
with aromatic lacy-edged leaves and daisy
flowers which are loved by bees. It is
excellent in the herb garden or flower
borders as its cheerful flowers bloom in late
summer when many others have died.

Feverfew derives its name from its ability

to bring down fevers; in one old tradition the herbalist had to pick the herb with the left hand and speak the name of the feverish patient while looking over his shoulder. In the days of Culpeper and Gerard, feverfew was valued for relieving ague, the old name for malaria, as well as colds and catarrh. It was used for menstrual problems, to protect against the plague, for bites of mad dogs, for nervous problems, particularly of hysterical women, to soothe pain and for convulsions.

Today, feverfew is famous as a remedy for headaches and migraine, best taken internally, eating the fresh leaves between two pieces of bread in a sandwich every day. If the fresh leaves are eaten alone, they may cause mouth ulcers. The bitter taste enhances digestion and liver function and thereby helps to clear toxins and heat from the body. Feverfew can also be used as an anti-inflammatory for arthritis, and to relieve nerve pain as in shingles and sciatica. Taken hot, it reduces fevers and acts as a decongestant for colds and catarrh. Due to its antihistamine action, it relieves allergies

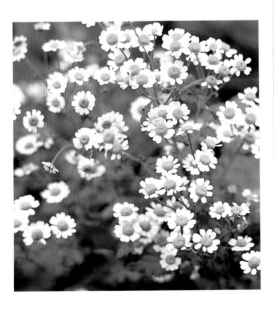

such as hay fever and asthma.
NB: Avoid in pregnancy.

How to Grow: Propagate by sowing seeds in spring, scattering them on the surface of well-drained soil and watering in. Likes full sun. Alternatively, divide plant in autumn. Self-seeds easily. Grows up to 90cm (3ft) and flowers in July and August.

Thymus vulgaris
THYME

Part used: Leaves and flowers
Contains: Tannins, bitters, essential oil, terpenes, flavonoids, saponins

Thyme is a much-loved small aromatic evergreen shrub, native to the Mediterranean where it can be found growing wild on warm dry rocky banks and heaths. The fragrant lilac or white flowers are loved by bees and impart a delicious flavour to honey. Thyme is widely grown for its culinary virtues and in various cultivated forms for garden decoration. It is also grown commercially for its wide use in medicines, antiseptic creams, mouthwashes and toothpastes.

Thyme's name comes from the Greek for 'smoke', as the Greeks burnt it both when making sacrifices to the gods and also as incense to dispel insects and contagion. The Romans slept on thyme to cure melancholy, and in the 16th century John Gerard said thyme was 'profitable for such as are ferfull melancholic and troubled in mind'. It was considered a strengthening tonic to the brain and an aid to increased longevity.

The volatile oils in thyme are highly antiseptic and, taken internally, support the

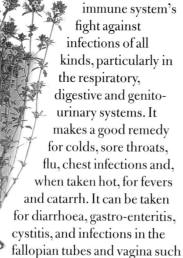

immune system's fight against infections of all kinds, particularly in the respiratory, digestive and genito-urinary systems. It makes a good remedy for colds, sore throats, flu, chest infections and, when taken hot, for fevers and catarrh. It can be taken for diarrhoea, gastro-enteritis, cystitis, and infections in the fallopian tubes and vagina such as thrush. It has a relaxant effect on the muscles in the bronchii, relieving asthma and dry hacking coughs, and in the digestive system, helping colic, wind, spastic colon and irritable bowel. It makes an excellent digestive herb, enhancing appetite and digestion and stimulating the liver, and has a strengthening effect on the nervous system. It has an antioxidant effect, protecting the body against the effects of the ageing process. Thyme can be taken for menstrual problems such as period pain, and as a cleansing diuretic to detoxify the body. Externally it can be used in liniments and lotions to relieve aching joints and muscular pain, to disinfect cuts and wounds and as a gargle for sore throats.

How to Grow: Propagate by sowing seeds in spring, by taking stem cuttings in summer, by dividing the roots in autumn or by layering older plants by mounding. Prefers well-drained, alkaline soil and full sun, and grows prostrate or upright to 30cm (1ft), flowering in summer. It is best to clip back after flowering and again in autumn to encourage bushy growth, otherwise thyme can become rather woody. May need replacing after 4 to 5 years.

Related plants with similar properties
T. o. citriodorus: Lemon-scented thyme
T. serpyllum: Wild thyme – good creeping plant for lawns
T. ×c.: Lemon thyme
T. ×c. 'Archers gold'
T. ×c. 'Aureus'
T. ×c. 'Golden king': variegated
T. ×c. 'Silver queen': silver– leafed
T. herba-barona: Caraway thyme
T. vulgaris 'Silver posie'

Tropaeolum majus
NASTURTIUM

Part used: Leaves, flowers, seeds
Contains: Glycoside (which hydrolyses to yield antibiotic sulphur compounds), iron, phosphates, potash, bitters, mineral salts

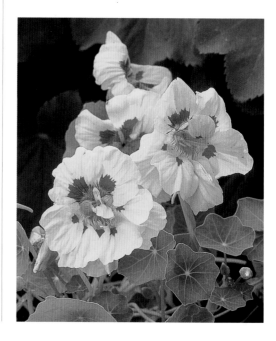

Nasturtiums are brightly coloured annuals indigenous to South America, with attractive flowers and peppery-flavoured leaves which are delicious in soups and salads. The leaves and flowers are high in vitamin C, minerals and trace elements, and the unripe seeds make a good substitute for capers.

Along with the gold of the Incas, the nasturtium was one of the acquisitions of the conquistadores in the 16th century. John Gerard was probably the first in England to get the seeds of 'this rare and fair plant' around 1597 and he grew it in his garden in Holborn. It was considered a rare treasure in Elizabethan England, valued for its beauty as well as its efficacy in treating scurvy.

The constituents of nasturtium resemble the mustard oil and sulphur compounds found in watercress (*Nasturtium officinale*). Taken internally, they both have bitter and pungent tastes, invigorating the digestion, improving appetite and absorption, and are excellent for treating weak digestion and sluggish livers. They stimulate liver, pancreas and gall-bladder action and the secretion of digestive enzymes and ensure healthy bowel function. Nasturtium also has a diuretic action which, together with its antimicrobial properties, makes it a good remedy for urinary infections and fluid retention. It is a good blood cleanser, improves the circulation and enhances immunity. It acts as a decongestant and is excellent when feeling tired and run down and prone to infections.

How to Grow: Nasturtiums are one of the easiest and most rewarding plants to grow from seeds, sown in spring and early summer. They like a sunny well-drained site and poor rather than fertile soil. Stems can creep or climb up to 3m (10ft). Flowers

through the summer. Dwarf, climbing and trailing varieties are ideal for most gardens. Atlantic hybrids have variegated leaves.

Valeriana officinalis
VALERIAN

Part used: Root and rhizome
Contains: Volatile oil, valepotriates, glycosides, alkaloids, choline, tannins, resins

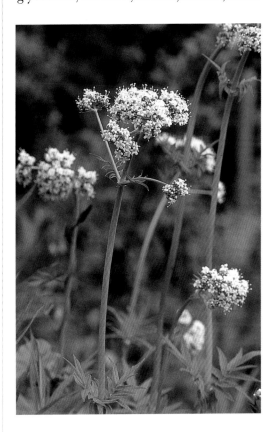

Valerian is a tall, hardy perennial, often to be found growing wild in ditches, woods and hedgerows. It has pretty fragrant pink flowers and strong-smelling roots which attract earthworms, so it is a good plant to grow in flower and vegetable gardens as well as the herb garden. The herb is said to intoxicate cats much like catmint, while legend says that the Pied Piper of Hamelin carried valerian to attract the rats towards the river.

Valerian was well known in the Middle Ages when the root was used as a medicine, as a spice and to perfume linen. It was esteemed as a remedy for epilepsy, hysteria, hypochondria, migraine, headaches and most problems affecting the nerves. Culpeper praised it as a good bruise herb, as well as to relieve coughs, fevers and the plague. Gerard said it was excellent for croup and convulsions. In the First World War valerian tincture was used for shell-shock and the strain on the nerves caused by air raids.

Today, valerian is highly valued as a sedative and tonic for the nervous system, excellent taken internally for anxiety, nervous tension, agitation, insomnia, nervous headaches and exhaustion. It strengthens and calms the heart and has the ability to lower blood pressure. The valepotriates which are mainly responsible for the calming effects of valerian are also relaxing to the smooth muscle throughout the body, so valerian can be used for many stress-related disorders such as muscle tension, colic, irritable bowel, period pain and headaches.

NB: Avoid large doses and prolonged use. Excessive doses may cause headaches, muscle spasm or palpitations.

How to Grow: Propagate by sowing seeds in spring in well-drained soil and full sun. Germination may be erratic. Alternatively, divide the plant in autumn. Grows up to 1.2-1.8m (4-6ft) tall and flowers in midsummer.

Harvest the root when the plant is two years old. It is a good idea to divide the plants every three years as they can easily get overcrowded.

Verbascum thapsus
MULLEIN

Part used: Leaves, flowers and root
Contains: Mucilage, volatile oil, saponins, resins, flavonoids, glycosides, gum

Mullein is an impressive biennial, its tall spikes of yellow flowers excellent in the back of herb or flower borders . Its soft, downy leaves were once used by country folk to line their shoes to keep their feet warm on cold days. The stems were dipped in tallow or suet and made good tapers or candles as far back as Roman days, while the leaves were used to wrap figs to keep them soft and moist. Roman women used the yellow dye from the flowers to colour their hair.

Since the days of the ancient Greeks mullein has been used to protect against infection, evil spirits and witches. Ulysses was said to have used mullein to protect himself against the sorcery of Circe. In Elizabethan times the leaves were carried to ward off epileptic attacks and water was distilled from the flowers as a remedy for gout. Mullein used to be cultivated widely in Ireland for its efficacy in treating tuberculosis. In America, the Native Americans boiled the leaves and applied them to painful joints and to relieve headaches.

Today, mullein is used internally, particularly for its soothing expectorant

MULLEIN (*Verbascum thapsus*)

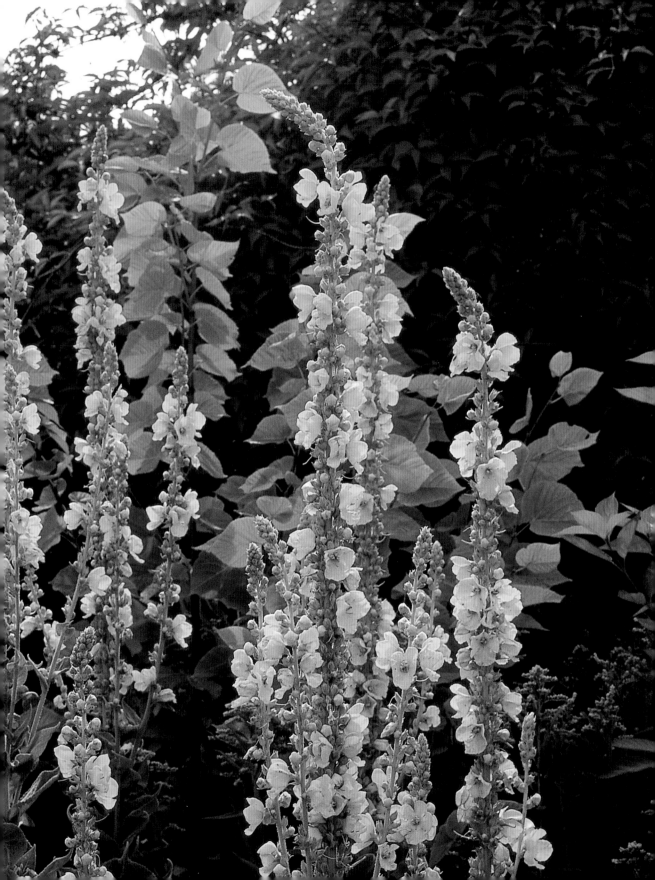

action in the respiratory system, excellent for harsh, irritating and dry coughs, sore throats and bronchitis. Its relaxing and antiseptic properties help to relieve asthma and croup as well as chest and throat infections. As a decongestant it helps clear phlegm, sinusitis and hay fever. Mullein also soothes cystitis and its diuretic action relieves fluid retention and increases elimination of toxins from the body. As a painkiller mullein can be used for headaches and neuralgia, arthritis and rheumatism. The flowers soaked in oil help to relieve earache.

How to Grow: Propagate by sowing seed in autumn in well-drained fertile soil. Press or water the seeds into the soil. In the first year mullein grows a large rosette of woolly leaves and the flowers arrive the next season. Self-seeds readily. The plant may attract mullein moth caterpillars which can devour most of the leaves. Grows 0.3-2m (1-6ft) high and flowers June to August.

Verbena officinalis

VERVAIN

Part used: Leaves and flowers
Contains: Glycosides, alkaloid, bitters, volatile oil, tannin

Vervain is a hardy perennial found growing wild in hedgerows and dry barren places. It has small, pretty lilac-coloured flowers on slender spikes and can be grown in pots or in clumps in the herb garden. It looks attractive grown by marsh mallow and white echinacea. It is cultivated extensively in Continental European countries, where vervain tea is very popular.

Despite its rather insignificant appearance, vervain was long considered to have magical properties, particularly by the Druids, who honoured it as sacred, a wizard's herb for divination and vital to magic potions. In Christian legends vervain was said to have grown at the foot of the cross and staunched the bleeding of Christ's wounds. Medieval magicians believed it was a panacea and could even confer immortality. Culpeper recommended it for 'female weaknesses', and other apothecaries prescribed it for jaundice, kidney disease, difficulty in pregnancy, heart disease and the plague.

Today, vervain is valued for its internal use as an excellent tonic to the nervous system, to calm the nerves, lift depression and support the body during stress. It can be thought of for most stress-related symptoms, such as headaches, indigestion, insomnia, high blood pressure, aches and pains and nervous exhaustion. Vervain also benefits the digestion, enhancing appetite and improving absorption. The bitters stimulate the liver and have a tonic action, relieving symptoms such as headaches, irritability and constipation. Taken hot it brings down fevers and taken cool it has a diuretic and detoxifying action.

It enhances milk supply in feeding mothers and regulates periods.

How to Grow: Propagate by sowing seeds in spring or autumn on the surface of well-drained soil in full sun. Press or water in the seeds. Grows 0.3-2m (1-6ft) and flowers July to September. Self-seeds easily.

Related plants
V. hastata: Blue /American vervain – for coughs, urinary stones, worms, nervous and skin problems
V. sticta: Wild blue vervain – for upset stomachs

Vinca minor/major
LESSER/GREATER PERIWINKLE

Part used: Flowering herb
Contains: Tannins, alkaloids, flavonoids, pectin

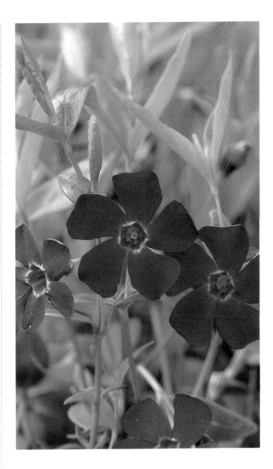

Periwinkle is a hardy evergreen spreading perennial, with sky-blue windmill-shaped flowers and shining leaves that make good ground cover throughout the winter. There is a cultivated silver variegated form as well as the two wild periwinkles found growing in woodlands and banks – lesser periwinkle, *V. minor*, and greater periwinkle, *V. major*, which has larger flowers and leaves.

Both greater and lesser periwinkle have been valued since antiquity for their medicinal benefits and for their part played in magic practices – periwinkle was commonly known as sorcerer's violet. Since the time of the ancient Greeks it has been used to protect against evil and to banish negativity. It was considered a vital ingredient in medieval love potions and the flowers were strewn at weddings. It was a good remedy for staunching bleeding cuts and wounds and for stopping diarrhoea and dysentery.

The astringent tannins in periwinkle have a binding quality – according to the Doctrine of Signatures this is indicated by their long creeping stems which resemble cords. Taken internally, they are excellent for curbing diarrhoea and dysentery and they protect the lining of the digestive tract from irritation and inflammation. Periwinkle will also stop bleeding internally and externally. It is often prescribed to reduce heavy periods, as well to stop bleeding of cuts and wounds. It will reduce catarrhal congestion and clear phlegm from the chest, and makes a good lotion for external use on varicose veins and haemorrhoids, and a gargle for sore throats. Since it has the ability to reduce blood sugar, it can be used in the treatment of diabetes.

How to Grow: Propagate by taking stem cuttings in autumn or divide roots in spring. Prefers fertile, moist soil and sun or shade. A good plant for growing along walls and fences where nothing much will grow in the shade. Grows 30-60cm (1-2ft) long and flowers March to May.

Related plants
V. rosea: Madagascan periwinkle – very helpful to diabetics as it reduces blood sugar. Two of its alkaloids have been used extensively to treat malignant tumours, as well as leukaemia and Hodgkin's disease.

Viola odorata

SWEET VIOLET

Part used: Flowers and leaves
Contains: Saponins, methyl salicylate, alkaloid, volatile oil, flavonoids, mucilage

This sweet little plant with its purple or white flowers and heart-shaped leaves is a hardy perennial found growing wild in woods and hedgerows in the spring. Violets have been widely popular for

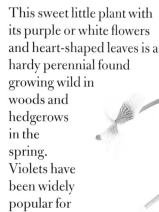

flavouring wines and syrups. They have also been used in perfumery and confectionary – crystallised leaves and flowers are still used to decorate cakes and puddings.

Violets were loved by the ancient Greeks, Romans and Persians, for use in their cosmetics, perfumery, flavouring and medicines. They would be woven into garlands to moderate anger and to ward off hangovers, and taken to cure headaches and induce sleep. Hippocrates also recommended them for melancholia, bad eyesight and inflammation of the chest. They were grown in medieval monastery gardens to protect against evil, while women made necklaces of violets to protect against deception, and put them in love potions.

Today, violets are used internally for their soothing and expectorant properties to relieve harsh irritating coughs and chest infections. Violet syrup is still popular as a children's cough syrup. Hot violet tea will bring down fevers and help clear congestion. Violets also soothe the gut and act as a gentle laxative. Their cooling properties will relieve heat and inflammation, while the salicylates are particularly useful for treating arthritis. In Chinese medicine violet flowers, leaves and root are used for hot swellings and cysts.

How to Grow: Propagate by sowing seeds in autumn or by planting rooted runners in autumn or spring in semi-shade in slightly acidic, moist soil. Flowers March to April. Keep young plants well watered in dry weather. Low growing 5-10cm (2-4in) high.

Viola tricolor

WILD PANSY

Part used: Leaves and flowers
Contains: Flavonoids, mucilage, tannins, salicylates, saponins, alkaloid

The pretty little heart-shaped flowers of this annual plant can be found growing wild in wheatfields and cultivated ground and flowering repeatedly from spring to autumn. It is an old favourite in English gardens and in old herbals it was called *Herba trinitas*, because each flower has three colours – purple, white and yellow.

Wild pansy is often called heartsease because of its ancient reputation for curing affairs of the heart – for easing the pain of separation and soothing a broken heart. It was also used in love potions, and Hippocrates used it as a cordial to lift the spirits and treat heart conditions. Gerard recommended it for ague, convulsions in children, inflammation in the chest and skin problems.

Wild pansy is still used internally for its soothing and expectorant properties to treat inflammatory chest problems, bronchitis, harsh irritating coughs, whooping cough, asthma and croup. Taken hot, it relieves catarrhal congestion and brings down fevers. Its soothing diuretic action relieves cystitis and fluid retention and has a detoxifying effect. It is often prescribed to cool the

system and clear skin conditions and its salicylates are helpful for treating arthritis and gout. It has a beneficial effect on the circulation, reducing blood pressure, strengthening blood vessels and helping to prevent arteriosclerosis.

How to Grow: Propagate by sowing seeds in spring and summer in rich, damp soil. Press seeds into soil and leave uncovered. Prefers semi-shade and grows 10-20cm (4-8in) high. Flowers from spring to autumn. Self-seeds freely. Deadhead flower heads to increase flowering and cut back leggy stems to encourage bushy growth.

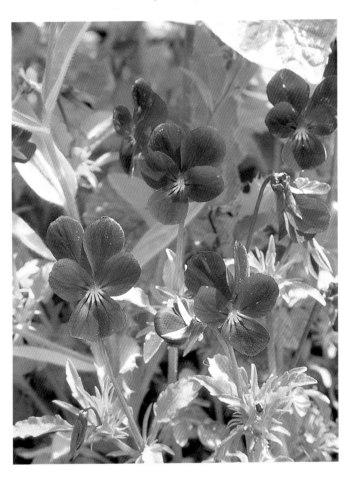

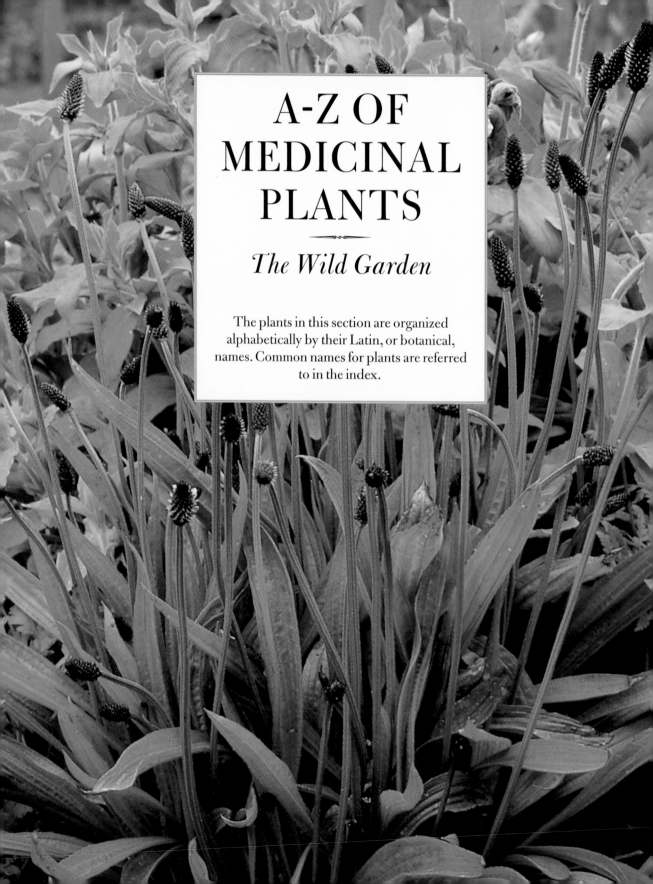

A-Z OF
MEDICINAL
PLANTS

The Wild Garden

The plants in this section are organized
alphabetically by their Latin, or botanical,
names. Common names for plants are referred
to in the index.

Agrimonia eupatoria
AGRIMONY

Part used: Leaves and flowers
Contains: Tannins, bitters, volatile oil, silica

Agrimony is a pretty, hardy perennial with slender long spikes of apricot-scented, pale yellow flowers, often found growing wild in summer hedgerows, meadows and waste ground.

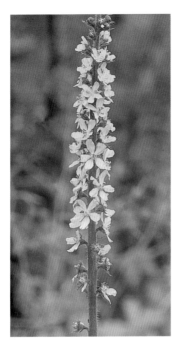

Its Latin name comes from the ancient Greek king Mithridates IV Eupator, who reigned 120 – 63 BC, a skilled herbalist who used agrimony to treat liver problems and poisoning. In medieval times agrimony was used to treat wounds, bruises and snakebites as well as to ward off evil.

Taken internally, agrimony makes an excellent digestive remedy, improving the secretion of digestive juices and of bile from the liver and gall bladder and enhancing the absorption of food. The astringent tannins protect the lining of the digestive tract from irritation and inflammation and help to heal inflammatory problems such as gastritis, colitis and peptic ulcers. Agrimony can be taken to relieve diarrhoea, and to treat liver and gall-bladder problems. It has a diuretic action, helping to cleanse toxins from the system, and is helpful when treating arthritis and gout. Agrimony makes a good gargle for sore throats and eyewash for inflammation of the eyes.

How to Grow: Propagate by sowing seeds from either February to May or August to November, in well drained soil and full sun. Alternatively, divide plants in autumn. Grows 15-60cm (6in-24in) tall and flowers from June to September.

Arctium lappa
BURDOCK

Part used: Roots, leaves, seeds
Contains: Roots – inulin, polyacetylenes, volatile oils, tannins, polyphenolic acids; seeds – fixed oils, bitter glycosides; leaves, arctiol, fulcinone, taraxasterol

Burdock is a handsome biennial plant with large rhubarb-like leaves, found growing wild in waste places and roadsides. It is grown in Japan as a vegetable and collected from the wild to eat by North American Indians. The root makes a nutritious vegetable and the peeled stalks can be cooked or candied like angelica.

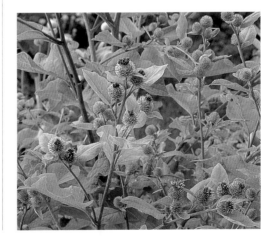

Since medieval times burdock has been valued medicinally for its cleansing and antiseptic properties. Apparently King Henry VIII was cured of syphilis with burdock and it was also used for leprosy. Culpeper recommended it for bites of snakes and mad dogs.

Taken internally, burdock root makes an excellent digestive and liver remedy and a mild laxative. Its mucilaginous fibres absorb toxins from the gut and carry them through the bowel to be eliminated. It is effective against bacterial and fungal infections and helps to re-establish normal bacterial population in the gut after using antibiotics and in candidiasis. Burdock also acts as a diuretic and makes an excellent remedy for chronic inflammatory conditions including arthritis, gout and skin diseases such as acne and psoriasis. It has been used traditionally for lowering blood sugar in diabetics and, taken as a hot tea, for fevers and eruptive infections like measles.

How to Grow: Burdock can be propagated by sowing seed in rich loamy soil in full sun or semi-shade and grows up to 1.8m (6ft) high.

Armoracia rusticana/Cochlearia armoracia

HORSERADISH

Part used: Fresh root
Contains: Sinigrin (a glycoside which yields mustard oil when mixed with water), vitamin C, resin, asparagin

Horseradish is a hardy perennial, with large dark-green leaves and very large tap roots which are well known as a condiment with an intensely pungent taste. Freshly grated horseradish makes an excellent flavouring, traditionally eaten with beef and fish and mixed with grated apple and cream to reduce its pungency. Young tender leaves can be chopped and eaten with green salads.

Horseradish has been valued as a medicine since at least Roman times and was one of the five bitter herbs the Jews ate during the feast of Passover. During the Middle Ages it was given to improve digestion and later Culpeper recommended it externally to relieve sciatica, gout, joint-ache and 'hard swellings of the spleen and liver'.

Taken internally, horseradish is a powerful stimulant, improving circulation and enhancing appetite, digestion and absorption. It has antibiotic properties similar to those of watercress, nasturtium and garlic, excellent for respiratory and urinary infections. The asparagin is a good diuretic and, by hastening elimination of toxins from the body, makes horseradish a good remedy for gout and arthritis. Its stimulating, decongestant and expectorant effects will help relieve coughs, colds, fevers, flu, catarrh, sinusitis and hay fever. Horseradish makes a good energy tonic, but is not recommended for symptoms characterised by heat, such as gastritis and peptic ulcers, or for people with thyroid problems.

How to Grow: Propagate by sowing seed in early spring or planting 20cm (8in) pencil-width root cuttings with a growing point in rich, moist, deep, well-manured soil and full sun. Keep watered in dry weather. Harvest roots in winter and store roots for replanting in damp sand. It is hard to eradicate the root once established so plant in a corner of the garden where it can spread. Grows 60-90cm (2-3ft) high. Flowers in midsummer though not every year.

Crataegus monogyra

HAWTHORN

Part used Flowers, leaves, berries
Contains: Saponins, glycosides, flavonoids, tannins, procyanidines, trimethylamine

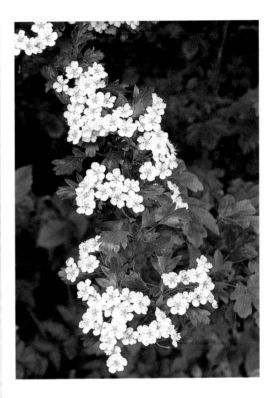

Hawthorn is a perennial shrub, a member of the rose family with a beautiful display of scented white blossoms in May and decorative red berries (haws) in autumn. Joseph of Arimathea is said to have introduced hawthorn to Britain when he arrived in Glastonbury in AD 60. He stuck his hawthorn staff into the ground and it grew into a tree.

Hawthorn has been traditionally associated with May Day and fertility customs, and has been connected with fertility and affairs of the heart since the days of the ancient Greeks and Romans, when it was present at wedding feasts and in nuptial chambers. Since medieval days hawthorn has been employed medicinally for heart and circulatory problems, fevers, gout and insomnia.

Taken internally, hawthorn is an excellent remedy for the heart and circulation, improving blood flow through the heart and arteries, reducing blood pressure and the build-up of deposits causing atherosclerosis. It regulates heart rhythm and is ideal for palpitations, arrhythmias, angina and degenerative heart disease as well as other circulatory problems elsewhere in the body. Hawthorn also has a relaxant effect, relieving anxiety and stress and promoting sleep. Its diuretic action helps reduce fluid retention and dissolve stones and gravel. It is a good digestive remedy and useful during menopause for night sweats and hot flushes.

How to Grow: Hawthorn is easily found growing wild. Seedlings can be bought, often by the hundred for hedging, at tree nurseries, to be planted from autumn to early spring. It will grow up to 4.5m (15ft) high in most soils and prefers semi-shade. Self-seeds freely.

Daucus carota

WILD CARROT

Part used: Herb, seed root
Contains: Herb and seed – volatile oil, alkaloid, root, vitamin C, B, B2, carotene, sugars, pectin, minerals

The wild carrot, also known as Queen Anne's lace, is the ancestor of the familiar domestic carrot. It is an attractive biennial and a member of the umbelliferae family, often found in hedgerows and stony or sandy ground near the sea. It was well known to the ancients, and was first mentioned by the Greeks in writings dating back to 500 BC.

The name *Daucus* comes from the Greek word meaning 'to burn', due to the pungent and stimulating qualities of carrots, particularly the seeds. These have been used for centuries to relieve flatulence, colic and dysentery and for a range of urinary complaints, particularly stones and gravel. The root was taken to improve appetite and

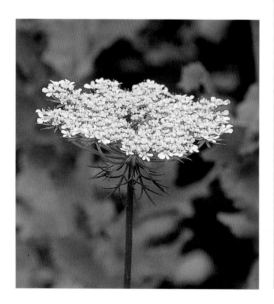

digestion, and tea made from the leaves was considered an excellent remdy for fluid retention and gout.

Today, the leaves and flowers of the wild carrot are used internally as an antiseptic diuretic for treating cystitis and prostatitis, and for a tendency to urinary stones and gravel. As a detoxifying remedy they are beneficial for gout and arthritis. Tea made from the seeds soothes and relaxes the digestive tract, relieving colic and indigestion, while the root has been used to expel worms from the intestines.

NB: Avoid seeds during pregnancy.

How to Grow: Propagate by sowing seeds in spring in light sandy soil and full sun. Grows 30-90cm (1-3ft) high and flowers in the second year in midsummer.

Galium aparine

CLEAVERS/CLIVERS

Part used: Leaves and flowers
Contains: Tannins, citric acid, asperuloside, saponins, coumarin

Cleavers is a common hedgerow perennial known for its long sticky stems and seeds which cling to anything they touch. It belongs to the "bedstraw" family, so-called for their strewing values in less hygienc times. The seeds used to be roasted and ground to make a substitute for coffee and the leaves were used to curdle milk as rennet does.

Taken as a soup, cleavers was an old wives' recipe for losing weight. In fact Culpeper said 'it is familiarly taken in broth to keep them lean and lank that are apt to

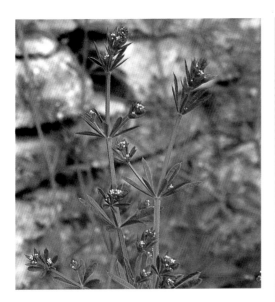

grow fat'. Gerard valued it as a cure for bites of spiders and snakes. A cooling drink of cleavers was traditionally taken each spring to 'clear the blood' and it has been eaten as a spring vegetable for similar cleansing purposes.

Cleavers still makes an excellent cleansing remedy if taken internally, clearing toxins and reducing heat and inflammation. It has diuretic properties and promotes lymphatic circulation, which makes it a good remedy for fluid retention, skin problems including eczema, psoriasis, acne and boils, urinary infections and stones, arthritis and gout. It can be taken for swollen lymph glands and lymphatic congestion and is said to have anti-tumour activity. Its cooling effect reduces fevers and helps to resolve eruptive infections such as measles and chicken pox, as well as inflammatory problems such as arthritis and cystitis. It improves digestion and stimulates the liver.

How to Grow: The wild seed easily propagates itself in cultivated land and waste places. Otherwise the seed can be sown in autumn or spring in most soils in sun or shade. Grows vigorously up to 3m (10ft) high and flowers through the summer.

Related plants
G. odoratum/asperula odorata: Sweet woodruff – a pretty, low-growing plant, used to scent linen and keep moths and fleas away, as well as to stimulate milk flow in nursing mothers

Glechoma hederacea/Nepeta hederacea
GROUND IVY

Part used: Leaves and flowers
Contains: Essential oil, tannins, bitters, resin

Ground ivy is a pretty little creeping perennial with purple-blue flowers, a familiar sight in wild grassland, hedgerows and woods. Its name comes from the resemblance of its leaves to those of the true ivy. While true ivy, which is highly aromatic, used to be woven into chaplets for the dead, ground ivy was used to decorate signs outside taverns, as it was popular in Saxon times for clarifying and flavouring ale, and was given the name alehoof.

Ground ivy has been popular as a medicine since earliest times. Galen in 2nd-century Greece recommended it for treating inflamed eyes, and later it was used for chronic bronchitis and nervous headaches, when the juice was sniffed up the nostrils. Gerard prescribed ground ivy for 'ringing noises of the ears and for those that are hard of hearing'.

Ground ivy is used internally today for its mild antiseptic and expectorant properties.

Taken hot, it also makes a good decongestant for colds, catarrh, congestive headaches and bronchial phlegm and brings down fevers. It has digestive properties and is gently astringent. Its diuretic action helps reduce fluid retention and clear toxins from the system.

How to Grow: Propagate by sowing seed in spring or autumn, covering lightly with soil. Prefers rich, fairly moist soil and sun, semi-shade or shade. It makes good ground cover, with stems reaching 10-30cm (4-12in) long. It flowers March to May.

Plantago major/Plantago minor/ Plantago lanceolata

PLANTAIN

Part used: Leaves
Contains: Mucilage, glycosides, tannins, silica

This familiar perennial is frequently found growing in lawns, footpaths, cultivated land and waste ground, easily recognised by its cylindrical spikes of seeds. The young leaves make a nutritious addition to salads.

Historically, plantain is famous as a wound healer and antidote to poisons. The Greeks and Romans used it for skin infections. Shakespare refers to it often as a healer, and it has been used as a folk remedy for toothache and earache.

Taken internally, plantain has a soothing action, particularly in the respiratory, digestive and urinary systems, relieving irritated and inflamed conditions such as colitis, gastritis, bronchitis, harsh coughs and cystitis. It has an astringent action, stemming bleeding and encouraging healing internally and externally, and is excellent for diarrhoea and catarrh. It can be taken for colds, sinus congestion and allergic conditions such as hay fever and asthma. It is antiseptic, cleansing and a good expectorant. The seeds of *P. psyllium,* mixed with water to form a gel, make an excellent bulk laxative. Externally, the fresh leaf applied to nettle, wasp and bee stings, and mosquito and flea bites, will bring relief.

How to Grow: Plantain will self-seed easily in most soils and grows up to 45cm (18in) high. It produces greenish-yellow flowers in summer followed by a spike of seeds.

Potentilla erecta/tormentilla

TORMENTIL

Part used: Root
Contains: Catechol-tannins, glycoside, red pigment, bitters, resin, gums

Tormentil is a pretty little perennial, with golden-yellow flowers, found growing wild among short grass, often on peaty soil.

Tormentil's name comes from the Latin *tormentum* meaning 'colic' or 'griping', as the plant was used in the past for intestinal pain and toothache. From the 16th century it was popular for its powerful astringent effect. Culpeper used it to stop bleeding, for

GROUND IVY (*Glechoma hederacea*)

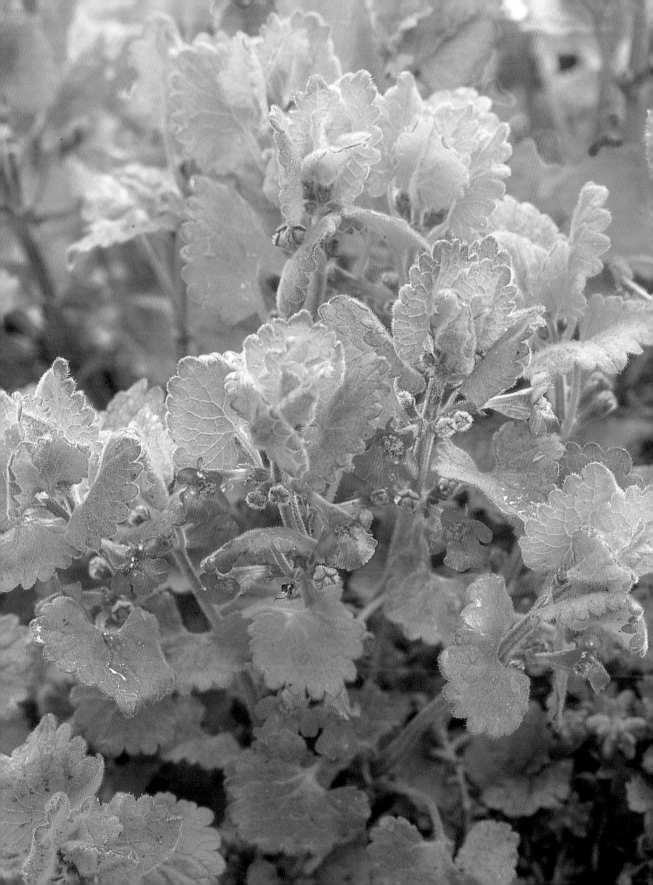

fevers and infections, and as an antidote to poisons. It was used for treating syphilis, diarrhoea, intermittent fevers, and ulcers.

Tormentil's astringent properties make it a good internal remedy for diarrhoea, gastro-enteritis and irritated conditions of the digestive tract. As a gargle it can be used for sore throats and as a mouthwash for infected gums and mouth ulcers. An external application to the skin will stem bleeding and speed healing of cuts, wounds,

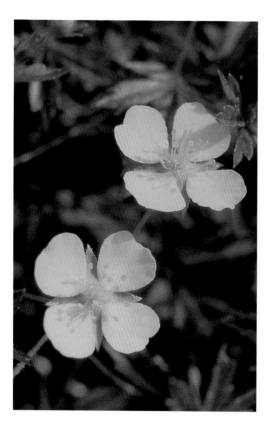

abrasions, burns and sunburn. It can be applied as a lotion to haemorrhoids and used as an eyewash for conjuctivitis.

How to Grow: Propagate by sowing seed in spring or autumn, covering the seed only lightly with soil. Will grow in most fertile soil and full sun. Grows 5-50cm (2-20in) and flowers from May to October.

Rumex crispus
YELLOW/CURLED DOCK

Part used: Root and leaf
Contains: Anthraquinone glycosides, tannins, iron

This inhabitant of hedgerows, meadows, ditches and roadsides is recognised by its yellowish roots and curled leaves. The leaves are known for relieving nettle stings and in the past were used for wrapping butter.

The roots, leaves and seeds have been valued medicinally since the days of the ancient Greeks, who recommended them for cleansing the body of toxins and aiding digestion. Gerard described dock's ability to stop the 'bloudie fluxe' and to ease stomach pains. Ointment made from the boiled roots, he said, 'helpeth the itch'. The seeds were used for dysentery and haemorrhages.

Today, dock root is still used for its detoxifying properties. Taken internally, its gentle laxative properties cleanse the bowel, while its astringent tannins check irritation and inflammation. The bitters stimulate the liver and benefit digestion. The diuretic properties increase elimination of toxins via the urinary system, making it useful for combatting fluid retention, cystitis, gout and arthritis. Dock is frequently used to clear skin problems, as well as to relieve chronic lymphatic congestion, anaemia, liver and digestive problems and constipation. It can also make a revitalising remedy for debility, headaches and low spirits. Externally, dock leaf or root tea makes a good lotion for skin

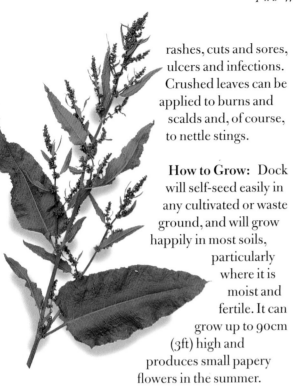

rashes, cuts and sores, ulcers and infections. Crushed leaves can be applied to burns and scalds and, of course, to nettle stings.

How to Grow: Dock will self-seed easily in any cultivated or waste ground, and will grow happily in most soils, particularly where it is moist and fertile. It can grow up to 90cm (3ft) high and produces small papery flowers in the summer.

Scrophularia nodosa

FIGWORT

Part used: Leaves and flowers
Contains: Saponins, flavonoids, resin, cardio-active glycosides

Figwort is an interesting perennial member of the foxglove family, found growing wild in Britain and America in woods, ditches and damp shady areas. Although the root tastes rather bitter it was once eaten as a vegetable – in fact it provided the only nourishment for a garrison in La Rochelle in France during a 13-month siege in 1628 and is known in French as *herbe de siège*.

The knobbly roots of figwort gave rise to its Latin name meaning 'swellings'. The old apothecaries called it *Ficaria major* because the roots were thought to resemble the ficus (Latin for 'fig'). Since they also looked like piles, the Doctrine of Signatures declared that they were an obvious cure for this problem. It was also thought to cure 'the king's evil' (a scrofulous skin condition caused by tuberculosis of the lymph nodes) and suppurating infective problems. Gerard said it 'keepeth a man in health' if worn around the neck or carried around. It was also believed to protect against the evil eye.

Today, figwort is predominantly used internally for its detoxifying properties in treatment of skin conditions. It stimulates lymphatic circulation as well as the peripheral blood circulation and thereby cleanses the tissues. It has a diuretic effect, hastening elimination of toxins via the kidneys, and is used for acne, boils, abscesses and other eruptive conditions. It also has a laxative effect, and the saponins, with their anti-inflammatory properties, help to relieve chronic inflammatory problems such as arthritis and gout. It is also used internally for swollen glands, mastitis and chronic tonsilitis and externally for wounds, burns, ulcers and inflamed skin conditions.

NB: Best used only with the advice of a qualified herbal practitioner.

How to Grow: Propagate by sowing seed in spring, in damp nutrient-rich soil, and semi-shade. Grows 0.6-1.2m (2-4ft) high and flowers from June to September. Self-seeds easily.

Stachys betonica

WOOD BETONY

Part used: Leaves and flowers
Contains: Tannins, saponins, alkaloids

Wood betony is a perennial woodland flower, found growing wild in woods and meadows, on heaths and moors and along country lanes. In the Middle Ages it was grown in apothecary and monastery gardens as it was considered almost a panacea, and in churchyards it was grown to protect against evil.

Medicinally, wood betony was highly praised in Roman times, being used for no fewer than 47 diseases. In medieval times it was considered effective treatment for jaundice, convulsions, gout, dropsy, headaches, aches and pains, palsy and bites of snakes and mad dogs.

The name betonica comes from the Celtic *ben* meaning 'head' and *tonic* meaning 'good' – as it was used to treat conditions associated with the head.

Today, wood betony is taken internally for the head, to relieve headaches from a variety of causes, including poor circulation, a sluggish liver and tension. It acts as a tonic to the nervous system and can be taken to relieve tension, anxiety, depression and lethargy. It soothes nerve pain, such as sciatica, as well as joint pain. It benefits the digestion and liver, and is useful in relieving indigestion, colic, wind, liver and gall bladder problems, as well as diarrhoea. It has a decongestant action when taken hot, and helps to throw off head colds. It also lowers blood sugar.

How to Grow: Propagate by sowing seeds in early spring or by dividing clumps in spring or autumn. Grows 30-60cm (1-2ft) high and flowers in June to September. Prefers fertile soil and light shade.

Stellaria media

CHICKWEED

Part used: Leaves and flowers
Contains: Saponins, mucilage, copper, tin, potash, salts, iron

Chickweed is a small annual plant which derives its Latin name from *stella* meaning 'star', due to its pretty, white star-shaped flowers. It has long been used for bird food as birds love it, and in winter it is one of their few sources of food. It can be eaten in salads and cooked like spinach, and, being rich in vitamins A and C and minerals including iron and copper, it is highly nutritious. Chickweed has been valued as a spring tonic and as a cooling remedy for hot inflammatory conditions. Culpeper recommended it 'for all heats and redness of the eyes', and it was used by country women to cool the body during fevers. It was rubbed onto arthritic joints to relieve pain and

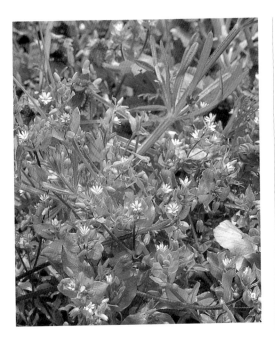

inflammation and drunk as tea to lose weight.

Today, chickweed, taken internally, makes a good cooling remedy for inflamed conditions of the digestive and respiratory tracts, such as gastritis, colitis, sore throats, asthma, bronchitis and pleurisy. Its diuretic action reduces fluid retention and helps eliminate toxins and heat from the system useful when treating arthritis, rheumatism and gout. Externally, chickweed cream or lotion will cool heat and rashes on the skin such as eczema, sunburn, boils and urticaria. The fresh leaves can be applied to burns and scalds, piles and ulcers, and as a drawing remedy to boils and abscesses.

How to Grow: Chickweed self-seeds easily. Low growing, it quickly spreads through open cultivated and waste ground to form a dense mat. Grows through most parts of the year, even when there is frost on the ground in early spring.

Taraxacum officinale
DANDELION

Part used: Leaves and root
Contains: Leaves – lutein, violaxanthin, bitters, vitamins A, B, C, D, potassium, iron; root – inulin, sterols, triterpenoids, bitters, pectin, glycosides, asparagin

Dandelion derives its common name from the French *dents de lion*, as the leaves were thought to resemble the jaw of a lion showing its teeth. The number of incisions on the toothed leaves of this perennial plant indicates the amount of sunlight it gets – with plenty of light it is deeply toothed, but in shady areas only slightly so , and will bloom only with sufficient sunlight. The young leaves are highly nutritious and delicious added to salads, and the roasted roots make an excellent coffee substitute.

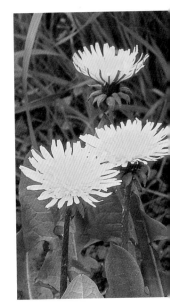

Dandelion was valued by the ancients as an antidote to poisons and for rheumatism, and it has long been said that if you drink a cup of dandelion tea daily you will never have rheumatism. The leaves were traditionally eaten in the spring as a cleansing tonic, and their diuretic properties earned dandelion the country names of pee-a-bed – in French *piss-en-lit*. Mothers would give their children dandelions to smell on May Day and hope they would not wet their beds for the rest of the year.

Today, dandelion is popular for internal

use as a bitter digestive and liver tonic, enhancing appetite and promoting digestion. By its action on the liver and its diuretic properties it is a gentle detoxifying remedy, aiding elimination of toxins via the kidneys. It can be used for skin problems, arthritis, gout, fluid retention and urinary infections, as well as for indigestion, liver and gall bladder problems. The white juice from the stems can be applied to warts.

How to Grow: Dandelion will seed itself easily in the garden and can be propagated by sowing but barely covering the seeds in spring, in most soils and full sun. Grows 5-30cm (2-12in) high and flowers from late spring to early autumn.

Urtica dioica

STINGING NETTLE

Part used: Leaves and flowers
Contains: Formic acid, histamine, acetylcholine, glucoquinones, chlorophyll, minerals, 5-hydroxytryptamine

The familiar nettle, much maligned for its cruel sting and tiresome tendency to invade our gardens, is a hardy perennial which was blessed by St Patrick as one plant put to more varied and useful purposes than any other. The young shoots and leaves are highly nutritious in spring soups and as a green vegetable, and have been used in beers, cheeses and shampoos. The fibrous leaves and stalks have been made into cloth, muslim nets and paper – in the First World War the Germans used nettles to make sail cloths, sacking and army uniforms.

Nettles were brought to England by the Romans under Julius Caesar. They used a particularly cruel nettle, *V. pilulifera*, to flog themselves to keep warm and to ward off illness caused by cold damp weather, such as colds, chest infections and arthritis. Stinging the skin in similar fashion to stimulate the circulation was recommended by Galen in the 2nd century AD as an aphrodisiac. Culpeper said nettles eaten in spring 'consume the plegmatic superfluities in the body of man that the coldness and moistness of winter hath left behind'.

Taken internally, nettles make an excellent detoxifying remedy and spring tonic. By stimulating the action of the liver and kidneys, they help to cleanse the body of toxins and wastes. By increasing excretion of uric acid through the kidneys, they help to relieve gout and arthritis. Their astringent properties reduce bleeding internally and externally; the fresh juice or tea can be applied to cuts and wounds, piles, burns and scalds, to stop bleeding and speed healing. They stimulate milk production in nursing mothers and have been used to regulate periods. When taken as a hot tea, nettles also help to clear catarrhal congestion and reduce fevers, and they make a good remedy for allergies such as eczema, asthma and hay fever.

How to Grow: Cultivation is rarely necessary as nettles will self-seed where they can. However, seeds can be sown or roots divided in spring and planted in good fertile soil.

Related plants
U. urens – annual nettle with smaller stems and leaves and similar uses

STINGING NETTLE (*Urtica dioica*)

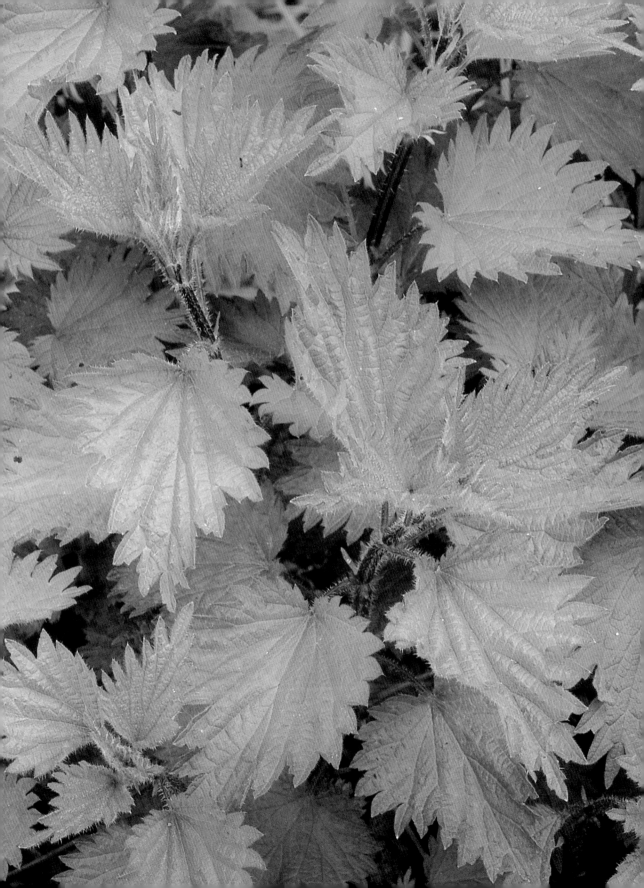

A quick reference guide to choosing herbal remedies for particular ailments.

HERBS	SKIN AND EYES	BONES, JOINTS, MUSCLES	CHILDREN'S AILMENTS	CIRCULATORY SYSTEM	DIGESTIVE SYSTEM	FIRST AID
Achillea millefolium Yarrow	Eczema. Skin repair.		Fevers, measles & chickenpox.	Varicose veins, haemorrhoids, poor circulation, high blood pressure.	Diarrhoea, wind, indigestion, gastritis, colitis.	Cuts, wounds, ulcers, burns. Antiseptic, anti-inflammatory. Promotes tissue repair.
Agrimonia eupatoria Agrimony	Irritated eyes.	Arthritis, gout.			Irritation, inflammation, gastritis, colitis, peptic ulcers, diarrhoea. Gall bladder & liver remedy.	
Alchemilla vulgaris Lady's mantle	Skin rashes.				Diarrhoea, gastritis, colitis, gastro-enteritis.	Rashes, cuts, abrasions.
Allium sativum Garlic			Ear infections, colds, coughs, fevers.	Heart problems, poor circulation. High blood pressure & cholesterol levels. Reduces tendency to clotting.	Stomach & bowel infections.	Antiseptic.
Allium schoenoprasm Chives				Anaemia.	Stimulates digestion, enhances absorption.	Antiseptic, antibacterial, antiviral, antifungal
Althea officinalis Marshmallow	Skin rashes. Draws out splinters.		Croup, dry coughs.		Heartburn, colitis, gastritis, irritable bowel.	Insect bites, scalds, burns, sunburn.

IMMUNE SYSTEM	MOTHER AND BABY	NERVOUS SYSTEM	REPRODUCTIVE SYSTEM	EAR, NOSE AND THROAT	URINARY SYSTEM	HERBS
Allergies, infections.			Regulates menstrual cycle. Relieves pain.	Fevers, colds, flu, catarrh.		*Achillea millefolium* Yarrow
				Sore throats.	Fluid retention.	*Agrimonia eupatoria* Agrimony
	Aids contractions, speeds recovery after birth. Avoid during pregnancy.		Heavy, painful or irregular periods. Genito-urinary infections, fibroids, pelvic inflammatory disease, vaginal infections.	Sore throats.	Urinary infections, fluid retention.	*Alchemilla vulgaris* Lady's mantle
Antibacterial, antiviral, antiparasitic, antifungal. Enhances immunity.		Invigorating tonic for debility.	Thrush.	Coughs, colds, catarrh, hay fever, asthma.	Cystitis, urinary infections.	*Allium sativum* Garlic
Enhances immunity. Combats infection.						*Allium schoenoprasm* Chives
	Teething.			Dry coughs, sore throat, asthma, bronchitis, inflamed gums.	Cystitis, irritable bladder, fluid retention.	*Althea officinalis* Marshmallow

HERBS	SKIN AND EYES	BONES, JOINTS, MUSCLES	CHILDREN'S AILMENTS	CIRCULATORY SYSTEM	DIGESTIVE SYSTEM	FIRST AID
Anemone pulsatilla Pasque flower	Eye infections.	Muscle spasm, pain.	Colic.		Colic.	
Anethum graveolens Dill		Muscle relaxant.	Colic, insomnia, restlessness.		Spasm, colic, wind, indigestion, nausea, constipation, diarrhoea.	
Anglica archanglica Angelica			Colic, fevers.	Poor circulation.	Nausea, indigestion, wind, colic.	
Apium graveolens Wild celery		Arthritis, rheumatism, gout.		Detoxicant.	Tonic for digestive system.	
Arctium lappa Burdock	Acne, psoriasis & other skin problems.	Arthritis, gout.	Measles, fevers, chickenpox.	Lowers blood sugar, detoxicant.	Constipation, indigestion. Liver remedy. Helps re-establish normal bacterial population in the bowel.	
Armoracia rusticana/Cochlea ria armoracia Horseradish		Arthritis, gout.		Poor circulation.	Poor appetite, weak digestion.	
Artemesia abrotanum Southernwood					Threadworms, roundworms. Stimulates digestion, improves liver function.	
Artemesia absinthium Wormwood	Skin problems.		Lowers fevers.		Worms, food poisoning. Stimulates appetite, promotes digestion & liver function.	

IMMUNE SYSTEM	MOTHER AND BABY	NERVOUS SYSTEM	REPRODUCTIVE SYSTEM	EAR, NOSE AND THROAT	URINARY SYSTEM	HERBS
Antibacterial.		Nerve tonic for insomnia, neuralgia, exhaustion, depression, irritability.	Period pain, PMT, menstrual headaches.	Colds, catarrh, coughs, ear infection, asthma.		*Anemone pulsatilla* Pasque flower
	Eases childbirth. Enhances milk supply in nursing mothers. Eases colic in babies.		Period pain. Regulates menstruation.	Dry coughs, asthma.		*Anethum graveolens* Dill
Enhances immunity, antibacterial, antifungal.	Avoid in pregnancy.	Strengthening tonic for nervous system.	Period pain, PMT. Regulates menstrual cycle.	Coughs, asthma, catarrh.		*Angelica archangelica* Angelica
Antiseptic.	Avoid in pregnancy.	Depression. Tonic for nervous system.			Fluid retention, cystitis.	*Apium graveolens* Wild celery
Enhances immunity, anti-inflammatory.					Fluid retention.	*Arctium lappa* Burdock
Antimicrobial.		Energy tonic.		Coughs, colds, flu, fevers, catarrh, sinusitis, hay fever.	Urinary infection, fluid retention.	*Armoracia rusticana/Cochlear ia armoracia* Horseradish
Antiseptic.	Increases efficiency of contractions in childbirth. Avoid in pregnancy.	Tonic for nervous system.	Promotes menstruation.			*Artemesia abrotanum* Southernwood
Enhances immunity. Aids convalescence.	Promotes contractions in childbirth. Avoid in pregnancy.	Detoxicant. Aids recovery from illness.	Painful or irregular periods.	Colds, flu, catarrh.		*Artemesia absinthium* Wormwood

HERBS	SKIN AND EYES	BONES, JOINTS, MUSCLES	CHILDREN'S AILMENTS	CIRCULATORY SYSTEM	DIGESTIVE SYSTEM	FIRST AID
Avena sativa Wild oats	Inflamed skin conditions.			Cardiovascular problems. Lowers blood cholestrol & blood sugar levels.	Constipation. Removes toxins from bowel.	
Calendula officinalis Marigold	Astringent.		Worms, fevers.	Improves lymphatic & blood circulation. Detoxicant.	Pelvic & bowel infections, diarrhoea. Enhances digestion, absorption, liver function.	Antiseptic. Cuts, abrasions, sores, ulcers, burns, cold sores. Staunches bleeding. Reduces infection.
Carduus benedictus/Cnicus benedictus Holy thistle			Diarrhoea, fevers.	Improves circulation.	Indigestion, diarrhoea, wind, poor appetite. Aids digestion & liver function.	
Chamomilla recutita/Matricari a chamomilla German chamomile *Anthemis nobilis* Roman chamomile	Skin disorders, e.g. eczema.	Arthritis, gout. Pain-relieving properties.	Hyperactivity, irritability.		Stress-related digestive symptoms.	Ulcers, sores, burns, scalds.
Cichorium intybus Chicory	Skin problems.			Regulates heart, reduces blood sugar level.	Constipation. Increases appetite. Promotes absorption & digestion. Stimulates liver & gall bladder function.	
Cimifuga racemosa Black cohosh		Muscular pain, arthritis & cramp.	Whooping cough.	Normalizes heart action, reduces high blood pressure, dilates arteries.	Colic.	
Coriandrum sativum Coriander	Conjunctivitis, skin rashes.	Arthritis	Fevers.		Enhances digestion & appetite. Improves absorption of nutrients.	
Crategus monogyra Hawthorn				High blood pressure, degenerative heart disease, cirulatory problems, atherosclerosis.	Aids digestion.	

IMMUNE SYSTEM	MOTHER AND BABY	NERVOUS SYSTEM	REPRODUCTIVE SYSTEM	EAR, NOSE AND THROAT	URINARY SYSTEM	HERBS
		Depression, anxiety. Aids withdrawal from tranquilizers & antidepressants.	Menopausal symptoms. Regulates hormones.			*Avena sativa* Wild oats
Candida, flu & herpes. Enhances immunity.	Do not take internally during pregnancy.		Period pain, menstrual congestion & heavy bleeding. Regulates periods. Menopausal problems.	Flu.		*Calendula officinalis* Marigold
Anti-tumor activity. Strengthens immune system.	Increases milk flow in nursing mothers. Avoid in pregnancy.	Headaches & lethargy. Tonic to nervous system.	Heavy periods, headaches, period pain.	Fever, catarrhal congestion.		*Carduus benedictus/Cnicus benedictus* Holy thistle
Enhances immune system. Antibacterial, antifungal & antihistamine.	Colic, teething & sleeping problems in babies. Eases contractions during childbirth.	Tension, anxiety, nervousness, over-sensitivity, pain, insomnia & headaches.	Period pain, pre-menstrual headaches, PMS. Thrush.	Colds, catarrh, hay fever, asthma.		*Chamomilla recutita/Matricaria chamomilla* German chamomile *Anthemis nobilis* Roman chamomile
Combats infection, antibacterial.					Fluid retention.	*Cichorium intybus* Chicory
Anti-inflammatory.	Relieves pain in childbirth.	Nerve pain, headaches. Anaesthetic.	Menopausal symptoms. Uterine pain, breast pain.	Asthma.		*Cimifuga racemosa* Black cohosh
		Stress-related disorders, e.g. gastritis, peptic ulcers, colic.	Period pain.	Sore throats.	Cystitis.	*Coriandrum sativum* Coriander
		Anxiety, stress & insomnia.	Menopausal symptoms, night sweats & hot flushes.		Fluid retention, stones, gravel.	*Crategus monogyra* Hawthorn

HERBS	SKIN AND EYES	BONES, JOINTS, MUSCLES	CHILDREN'S AILMENTS	CIRCULATORY SYSTEM	DIGESTIVE SYSTEM	FIRST AID
Cynara scolymus Globe artichoke				High cholesterol & triglyceride levels. Arteriosclerosis.	Heartburn, nausea, poor appetite, liver insufficiency, jaundice.	
Daucus carota Wild carrot		Arthtritis, gout.		Detoxicant.	Indigestion, colic, worms.	
Echinacea angustfolia/ purpurea/pallida Purple cone flower	Boils, abscesses.	Arthritis, gout.	Fevers, measles, mumps & chickenpox.	Enhances circulation.		
Erica vulgaris/Calluna vulgaris/tetralix/ cinerea Heather	Skin problems, e.g. acne	Arthritis, gout, muscle tension.		Detoxicant.		
Eupatorium purpureum Joe Pye weed		Arthritis, gout.		Detoxicant.		
Filipendula ulmaria Meadowsweet		Arthritis, rheumatism.	Colic & fevers. Eruptive infections, e.g. measles, chickenpox.	Atherosclerosis. Detoxicant.	Acidity, gastritis, ulcers, wind, diarrhoea, enteritis & colic.	
Foeniculum vulgare Fennel	Sore eyes.		Colic.		Wind, nausea, indigestion, heart-burn & colic.	
Fragaria vesca Wild strawberry	Skin blemishes. Whitens teeth.	Gout.	Fevers.		Diarrhoea. Stimulates liver, enhances digestion.	Stems bleeding.

IMMUNE SYSTEM	MOTHER AND BABY	NERVOUS SYSTEM	REPRODUCTIVE SYSTEM	EAR, NOSE AND THROAT	URINARY SYSTEM	HERBS
					Fluid retention, urinary infections.	*Cynara scolymus* Globe artichoke
Antiseptic.	Avoid seeds in pregnancy.				Cystitis, prostatis, urinary stones, gravel.	*Daucus carota* Wild carrot
Infections, allergies, candida. Enhances immunity. Anti-bacterial, anti-fungal, antiviral & anti-inflammatory.		Local anaesthetic.	Pelvic inflammatory disease.	Sore throats, colds, flu, chest infections, glandular fever.		*Echinacea angustfolia/purpur ea/pallida* Purple cone flower
		Anxiety & insomnia.			Urinary infections, fluid retention.	*Erica vulgaris/Calluna vulgaris/tetralix/ci nerea* Heather
			Menstrual pain, pelvic inflammatory disease.		Urinary infections, stones, gravel, fluid retention. Prostate problems.	*Eupatorium purpureum* Joe Pye weed
Antiseptic & anti-inflammatory.		Headaches & neuralgia. Anaesthetic.			Fluid retention, kidney stones & gravel.	*Filipendula ulmaria* Meadowsweet
	Aids milk production in nursing mothers. Relieves babies' colic. Avoid in pregnancy.		Period pain, menopausal symptoms. Regulates menstrual cycle.		Fluid retention, cellulite, urinary infections.	*Foeniculum vulgare* Fennel
				Sore throats.	Fluid retention.	*Fragaria vesca* Wild strawberry

HERBS	SKIN AND EYES	BONES, JOINTS, MUSCLES	CHILDREN'S AILMENTS	CIRCULATORY SYSTEM	DIGESTIVE SYSTEM	FIRST AID
Fumaria officinalis Fumitory	Skin problems, e.g. psoriasis, eczema, acne. Increases sweating.			Detoxicant.	Laxative, liver tonic & digestive problems.	
Galium aparine Cleavers/clivers	Skin problems, e.g. eczema, acne & boils.	Arthritis & gout.	Fevers, chickenpox & measles.	Detoxicant, promotes lymphatic circulation.	Improves digestion, stimulates liver.	
Glechoma hederacea/nepeta Ground ivy	Inflamed eyes.		Fevers.	Detoxicant.	Aids digestion, diarrhoea.	Cuts, abrasions. Stems bleeding.
Glycyrrhiza glabra Liquorice		Arthritis.	Allergies.	Lowers cholesterol.	Liver remedy, ulcers, irritation, inflammation, acidity, heartburn & indigestion.	
Hammamelis virginiana Witch hazel	Skin problems, inflamed eyes & greasy skin.			Varicose veins, haemorrhoids & phlebitis.	Colitis, dysentry, diarrhoea.	Burns, bruises, sprains, insect bites. Stems bleeding.
Helianthus annuus Sunflower		Arthritis, gout, rhematism.	Fevers.			
Humulus lupulus Hops		Muscle tension.			Stress-related problems, e.g. irritable bowel, liver problems & diverticultis.	
Hypericum perforatum St John's wort				Varicose veins.		Burns, cuts, wounds, sores, ulcers, sprains, bruises, sunburn.

IMMUNE SYSTEM	MOTHER AND BABY	NERVOUS SYSTEM	REPRODUCTIVE SYSTEM	EAR, NOSE AND THROAT	URINARY SYSTEM	HERBS
	Cradle cap.				Fluid retention.	*Fumaria officinalis* Fumitory
Anti-inflammatory.				Swollen glands.	Cystitis, fluid retention.	*Galium aparine* Cleavers/clivers
Anti-microbial.				Sore throats, colds, flu, catarrh, congestive headaches, chest infections.	Fluid retention.	*Glechoma hederacea/nepeta* Ground ivy
Allergies & inflammatory allergies.		Improves resistance to stress.	Menopausal symptoms.	Coughs, asthma, chest infections.		*Glycyrrhiza glabra* Liquorice
	Tones uterus after miscarriage or childbirth.		Uterine prolapse, heavy periods.	Chronic catarrh.		*Hammamelis virginiana* Witch hazel
Enhances immunity.				Asthma, sore throats, colds, coughs.	Fluid retention.	*Helianthus annuus* Sunflower
	Colic.	Anxiety, stress, pain & insomnia.	Menopausal problems.			*Humulus lupulus* Hops
Enhances immunity. Antiviral & antibacterial.		Tension, anxiety, depression, SAD, nerve pain.	Menopausal problems.			*Hypericum perforatum* St John's wort

HERBS	SKIN AND EYES	BONES, JOINTS, MUSCLES	CHILDREN'S AILMENTS	CIRCULATORY SYSTEM	DIGESTIVE SYSTEM	FIRST AID
Hyssopus officinalis Hyssop	Increases sweating.		Fevers.	Stimulates circulation, detoxicant.	Constipation, colic & indigestion.	
Inula helenium Elecampane	Skin infections, e.g. scabies, herpes.		Fevers.	Stimulates circulation.	Worms. Stimulates liver, aids digestion.	Antiseptic wash for cuts, wounds.
Jasminum grandiflorum/ Jasminum officinalis Jasmine				Improves lymphatic circulation.	Colic.	
Laurus nobilis Sweet bay		Arthritis, rheumatism.		Stimulates circulation.	Poor appetite, indigestion, wind, gastro-intestinal infections.	
Lavendula officinalis Lavender	Acne. Stimulates tissue repair, minimizes scar formation.	Muscle tension.	Fevers.	Detoxicant.	Wind, nausea, indigestion, colic, stress-related problems, bowel problems.	Burns, scalds, sores, ulcers. Insect repellent.
Leonurus cardiaca Motherwort				Palpitations. Lowers blood pressure.		
Levisticum officinalis Lovage			Fevers.	Promotes circulation. Detoxicant.	Aids digestion.	
Linum usitatissimum Flax/Linseed				Thrombosis. Detoxicant. Lowers blood cholesterol & pressure.	Gastritis, enteritis, colitis. Laxative.	

IMMUNE SYSTEM	MOTHER AND BABY	NERVOUS SYSTEM	REPRODUCTIVE SYSTEM	EAR, NOSE AND THROAT	URINARY SYSTEM	HERBS
Enhances immunity. Anti-microbial.		Tonic for nervous system.		Colds, flu, catarrh, chest infections, asthma. Expectorant.		*Hyssopus officinalis* Hyssop
Antibacterial & antifungal.				TB, catarrh, colds, asthma, bronchitis & other chest infections.		*Inula helenium* Elecampane
Antiseptic.	Soothes pain & eases contractions during childbirth.	Stress, headaches, anxiety.	Period pain, PMS, heavy periods, genito-urinary infections, e.g. salpingitis.	Colds, catarrh, bronchial congestion.	Cystitis.	*Jasminum grandiflorum/ Jasminum officinalis* Jasmine
Enhances immunity.				Bronchial catarrh, coughs, chest infections.		*Laurus nobilis* Sweet bay
Antimicrobial, enhances immunity.		Anxiety, stress, nervousness, headaches, nerve pain, insomnia, depression.		Sore throats, flu, colds, chest infections, catarrh.		*Lavendula officinalis* Lavender
	Soothes tension surrounding child-birth. Relieves pain during childbirth. Avoid in pregnancy until last trimester.	Relaxant, reduces stress & anxiety.	Period pain, menopausal symptoms.			*Leonurus cardiaca* Motherwort
				Catarrh.	Fluid retention.	*Levisticum officinalis* Lovage
				Coughs, sore throats.	Cystitis, irritable bladder.	*Linum usitatissimum* Flax/Linseed

HERBS	SKIN AND EYES	BONES, JOINTS, MUSCLES	CHILDREN'S AILMENTS	CIRCULATORY SYSTEM	DIGESTIVE SYSTEM	FIRST AID
Lonicera pericilymenum Wild honeysuckle		Arthritis, rheumatism, muscular aches.	Croup, asthma, whooping cough.	Detoxicant.	Laxative.	
Melissa officinalis Lemon balm	Eczema.		Colic, fevers, childhood infections, e.g. mumps.		Irritation, inflammation & stress-related digestive problems. Aids digestion.	
Mentha piperita Peppermint	Inflammatory skin problems.		Fevers.	Stimulates circulation.	Nausea, vomiting, diarrhoea, colic, indigestion, bowel problems.	Travel sickness.
Nepeta cararia Catmint	Rashes.	Muscle tension.	Fevers, measles & chickenpox.	Stimulates circulation.	Upset stomachs, indigestion, inflammatory bowel problems, diarrhoea.	Cuts, bites, burns, scalds, bruises. Antiseptic. Stops bleeding.
Ocimum basilicum Basil		Muscle tension.			Cramp, diarrhoea, constipation, nausea, indigestion.	Minor cuts, grazes, bites, stings.
Oenothera biennis Evening primrose	Skin erruptions, eczema.	Arthritis.	Hyperactivity, allergies.	High blood pressure, high cholesterol, coronary artery disease.	Soothes irritation. Aids regeneration of damaged liver.	
Oreganum marjorana Sweet marjoram		Arthritis, gout, muscular pain.	Fevers.	Improves circulation. Detoxicant.	Digestion, colic, abdominal pain, indigestion.	
Passiflora incarnata Passionflower		Muscular aches, cramps.		High blood pressure.	Colic & stress-related problems.	

IMMUNE SYSTEM	MOTHER AND BABY	NERVOUS SYSTEM	REPRODUCTIVE SYSTEM	EAR, NOSE AND THROAT	URINARY SYSTEM	HERBS
Anti-inflammatory, antimicrobial.		Stress-related problems, headaches, anxiety.		Flu, asthma, bronchitis, chest infections. Expectorant.	Fluid retention.	*Lonicera pericilymenum* Wild honeysuckle
Infection, e.g. mumps, herpes. Allergies.	Eases pain during childbirth.	Depression, anxiety & insomnia.	Period pain, PMS.	Catarrhal congestion, hay fever.		*Melissa officinalis* Lemon balm
Enhances immunity, anti-microbial.		Lethargy. Increases energy.	Period pain.	Catarrh, colds, flu, herpes, chest infections.		*Mentha piperita* Peppermint
	Wind, colic in babies.	Stress-related problems.	Period pain, PMS.	Coughs, asthma, bronchitis, Decongestant, expectorant.		*Nepeta cararia* Catmint
Antiseptic, helps fight off infections.		Nerve tonic, nerve pain, anxiety, tension & depression.		Colds, flu, catarrh, coughs, sore throats, asthma.		*Ocimum basilicum* Basil
Allergies. Enhances immunity.		Nervous tension, migraine.	Hormonal problems, PMS, menopausal symptoms.	Asthma.		*Oenothera biennis* Evening primrose
Enhances immunity, antibacterial & antiviral.	Avoid in pregnancy.	Anxiety, tension, insomnia, depression.	Period pains, PMS.	Colds, sore throats, chest infections, flu, catarrh, herpes.	Fluid retention.	*Oreganum marjorana* Sweet marjoram
	Colic, croup in babies.	Headaches, pain, neuralgia, anxiety, insomnia.Relaxant & sedative.	Period pain.	Coughs, asthma, nervous coughs.		*Passiflora incarnata* Passionflower

HERBS	SKIN AND EYES	BONES, JOINTS, MUSCLES	CHILDREN'S AILMENTS	CIRCULATORY SYSTEM	DIGESTIVE SYSTEM	FIRST AID
Petroselinum crispus Parsley		Arthritis, gout.		Tonic for anaemia. Stimulates circulation. Detoxicant.	Colic, indigestion & wind. Stimulates appetite, improves digestion & absorption.	
Plantago major Greater plantain					Constipation, gastritis, colitis.	Nettle, wasp & bee stings, mosquito & flea bites. Stems bleeding.
Polygonum bistorta Bistort				Haemorrhoids, varicose veins, varicose ulcers.	Diarrhoea, dysentry, colitis.	Stems bleeding, e.g. nosebleeds, bleeding gums, mouth ulcers.
Potentilla erecta/ tormentilla Tormentil	Conjunctivitis.			Haemorrhoids.	Diarrhoea, gastroenteritis, irritated digestive tract.	Cuts, wounds, burns, sunburn. Stems bleeding.
Primula veris Cowslip	Skin problems.	Arthritis, gout.	Fevers.			
Pulmonaria officinalis Lungwort	Cuts, wounds, burns, scalds, sores, ulcers.			Haemorrhoids, varicose veins.		Cuts, wounds, bleeding, burns, scalds.
Rosa sp. Rose	Skin rashes.		Fevers.	Detoxicant.	Re-establishes bacterial population.	
Rosmarinus officinalis Rosemary		Arthritis, rheumatism.	Fevers.	Increases circu-lation, particularly to the head.	Diarrhoea. Digestive tonic, stimulates liver & gall bladder.	Stems bleeding.

IMMUNE SYSTEM	MOTHER AND BABY	NERVOUS SYSTEM	REPRODUCTIVE SYSTEM	EAR, NOSE AND THROAT	URINARY SYSTEM	HERBS
Combats infection.	Aids childbirth, increases milk in nursing mothers. Avoid in pregnancy.	Anxiety, lethargy, depression, headaches, migraine.		Asthma.	Infections, fluid retention, irritable bladder. Avoid in kidney disease.	*Petroselinum crispus* Parsley
Allergies. Enhances immunity.				Hay fever, asthma, irritating coughs, bronchitis, catarrh.	Infection, e.g. cystitis.	*Plantago major* Greater plantain
			Heavy periods.	Catarrhal, sore throats, congestion.		*Polygonum bistorta* Bistort
Conjunctivitis, infected gums, mouth ulcers.				Sore throats, infected gums, mouth ulcers.		*Potentilla erecta/ tormentilla* Tormentil
Anti-inflammatory.		Nerve tonic. Headaches, anxiety, tension, insomnia, depression.		Colds, sore throats, catarrh, coughs, flu. Expectorant.		*Primula veris* Cowslip
				Coughs, catarrh, bronchial irritation.		*Pulmonaria officinalis* Lungwort
Enhances immunity, anti-inflammatory.	Avoid in pregnancy.	Nerve tonic. Anxiety, depression.	Painful & heavy periods, pelvic congestion. Enhances sexual desire.	Colds, flu, sore throats, catarrh, chest infections.		*Rosa* sp. Rose
Enhances immunity, antimicrobial.		Depression, anxiety, poor memory, headaches, migraines. Nerve tonic.	Heavy periods.	Colds, flu, catarrh, sore throats, chest infections.	Fluid retention.	*Rosmarinus officinalis* Rosemary

HERBS	SKIN AND EYES	BONES, JOINTS, MUSCLES	CHILDREN'S AILMENTS	CIRCULATORY SYSTEM	DIGESTIVE SYSTEM	FIRST AID
Rubus idaeus Raspberry			Fevers.	Anaemia.	Diarrhoea.	Wounds, ulcers, burns, scalds. Stems bleeding.
Rumex crispus Yellow/Curled dock	Skin problems, eczema, psoriasis, acne.	Arthritis, gout.		Anaemia, lymphatic congestion. Detoxicant.	Irritation, inflammation, constipation. Liver remedy.	Cuts, sores, ulcers, infections, burns, scalds, nettle stings & rashes.
Salvia officinalis Sage	Stops sweating.	Arthritis, gout.	Fevers.	Detoxicant.	Colic, indigestion. Stimulates appetite, enhances digestion. Liver tonic.	Cuts, wounds, burns, sores, ulcers, sunburn.
Salvia sclarea Clary sage	Eye irritation. Excessive perspiration.		Colic.		Indigestion, pain & spasm in the digestive tract.	
Sambucus nigra Elder	Skin problems.	Arthritis, gout.	Fevers, colds, measles, chicken pox.	Detoxicant, causes sweating, increases circulation.		Sunburn.
Saponaria officinalis Soapwort	Skin problems, e.g. psoriasis, acne, boils, eczema.	Arthritis, gout, rheumatism.		Detoxicant.	Constipation. Liver remedy.	
Scrophularia nodosa Figwort	Skin conditions, e.g. acne, boils.	Arthritis, gout.	Measles, chicken pox.	Stimulates lymphatic & blood circulation. Detoxicant.	Constipation.	Wounds, burns, ulcers.
Scutellaria laterifolia Virginian skullcap		Tense, aching muscles. Arthritis.	Fevers.	Palpitations.	Digestive problems.	

IMMUNE SYSTEM	MOTHER AND BABY	NERVOUS SYSTEM	REPRODUCTIVE SYSTEM	EAR, NOSE AND THROAT	URINARY SYSTEM	HERBS
	Helps contractions. in childbirth. Heals womb. Stimulates milk in nursing mothers.			Sore throats.	Fluid retention.	*Rubus idaeus* Raspberry
	Avoid in pregnancy.	Debility, head-aches, depression.			Fluid retention, cystitis.	*Rumex crispus* Yellow/ Curled dock
Antibacterial, antifungal.	Avoid in pregnancy and while breast-feeding.		Irregular, scanty or painful periods. Menopausal problems, e.g. night sweats.	Colds, flu, fevers, sore throats, chest infections.	Fluid retention.	*Salvia officinalis* Sage
	Pain & spasm in uterus. Soothes contractions during childbirth. Post-natal depression. Avoid in pregnancy.	Insomnia, head-aches, depression, exhaustion. Nerve tonic, relaxant.	Period pain, menopausal symptoms	Asthma, harsh coughs.		*Salvia sclarea* Clary sage
			Diuretic, detoxicant.	Colds, flu, sore throats, catarrh, coughs, asthma.	Fluid retention.	*Sambucus nigra* Elder
Anti-inflammatory.				Expectorant		*Saponaria officinalis* Soapwort
Anti-inflammatory.	Mastitis.			Swollen glands, tonsilitis.	Fluid retention.	*Scrophularia nodosa* Figwort
		Anxiety, headaches, depression. Soothes nerves, releases tension. Promotes sleep.	Period pain.			*Scutellaria laterifolia* Virginian skullcap

HERBS	SKIN AND EYES	BONES, JOINTS, MUSCLES	CHILDREN'S AILMENTS	CIRCULATORY SYSTEM	DIGESTIVE SYSTEM	FIRST AID
Silybum marianis Milk thistle				Detoxicant.	Liver diseases, alcohol-induced cirrhosis, jaundice, chronic liver disease, hepatitis, liver damage.	Travel sickness.
Solidago virgaurea Goldenrod	Wounds, ulcers.	Arthritis, gout.	Fevers.	Detoxicant.	Diarrhoea, colic, nausea.	Cuts, wounds, ulcers. Stems bleeding.
Stachys betonica Wood betony		Joint pain.		Lowers blood sugar. Improves circulation.	Diarrhoea, indigestion, gall bladder problems sluggish liver, colic, wind.	
Stellaria media Chickweed	Eczema, urticaria, ulcers, boils, abscesses.	Arthritis, gout, rheumatism.		Haemorrhoids, varicose ulcers.	Gastritis, colitis.	Sunburn, burns, scalds, rashes.
Symphytum officinale Comfrey	Skin problems.	Arthritis, gout. Speeds repair of connective tissue, cartilage, bone & collagen.			Gastritis, peptic ulcers, diarrhoea, dysentry, ulcerative colitis.	Stems bleeding. Cuts, wounds, burns, scalds, sores, ulcers.
Tanacetum parthenium Feverfew		Arthritis.	Fevers.	Detoxicant.	Enhances digestion & liver function.	
Taraxacum officinale Dandelion	Skin problems, e.g. warts.	Arthritis, gout.		Detoxicant.	Poor appetite, weak digestion, liver & gall bladder problems.	
Thymus vulgaris Thyme		Aching joints, muscular pain.	Fevers, whooping cough, asthma.	Detoxicant, stimulates circulation.	Diarrhoea, wind, gastroenteritis, spastic colon, irritable bowel.	Cuts & wounds. Antiseptic.

IMMUNE SYSTEM	MOTHER AND BABY	NERVOUS SYSTEM	REPRODUCTIVE SYSTEM	EAR, NOSE AND THROAT	URINARY SYSTEM	HERBS
						Silybum marianis Milk thistle
			Period pain.	Catarrhal congestion.	Infections, stones, fluid retention.	*Solidago virgaurea* Goldenrod
		Anxiety, neuralgia pain, e.g. headaches, depression, tension, lethargy. Nerve tonic.		Catarrh, colds.		*Stachys betonica* Wood betony
Anti-inflammatory.	Sore nipples.			Sore throats, asthma, bronchitis, pleurisy.	Fluid retention.	*Stellaria media* Chickweed
Protects against infection & inflammation.				Sore throats, coughs.	Cystitis, irritable bladder.	*Symphytum officinale* Comfrey
Allergies. Anti-inflammatory.	Avoid in pregnancy.	Migraines, headaches, shingles, sciatica.		Antihistamine, colds, catarrh.		*Tanacetum parthenium* Feverfew
					Fluid retention, infections.	*Taraxacum officinale* Dandelion
Enhances immunity, antimicrobial.	Avoid in pregnancy.	Nerve tonic.	Infections in fallopian tubes & vagina e.g. thrush. Period pain.	Asthma, colds, sore throats, flu, chest infections, fever, catarrh.	Cystitis, urinary infections.	*Thymus vulgaris* Thyme

HERBS	SKIN AND EYES	BONES, JOINTS, MUSCLES	CHILDREN'S AILMENTS	CIRCULATORY SYSTEM	DIGESTIVE SYSTEM	FIRST AID
Tropaolum majus Nasturtium				Improves circulation, detoxicant.	Improves digestion, liver function, weak digestion & constipation.	
Urtica dioica Stinging nettle	Eczema.	Arthritis, gout.	Fevers.	Haemorrhoids. Detoxicant.	Sluggish liver.	Cuts, wounds, burns, scalds. Stems bleeding.
Valeriana officinalis Valerian		Muscle tension.		Calms heart, lowers blood pressure.	Irritable bowel, colic & spasm.	
Verbascum thapsus Mullein		Arthritis, rheumatism.	Asthma, croup, earache.			
Verbena officinalis Vervain			Fevers.	High blood pressure.	Constipation & stress-related digestive problems. Enhances appetite, digestion & absorption.	
Vinca minor/ major Lesser/ Greater periwinkle				Varicose veins, haemorrhoids. Reduces blood sugar.	Diarrhoea, dysentry. Protects digestive tract.	Cuts & wounds. Stems bleeding.
Viola odorata Sweet violet		Arthritis.	Fevers. Good children's cough syrup.		Laxative, soothes inflammation.	
Viola tricolor Wild pansy	Skin problems.	Arthritis, gout.	Fevers, whooping cough, croup.	Helps prevent arterio-sclerosis, strengthens blood vessels. High blood pressure. Detoxicant.		

IMMUNE SYSTEM	MOTHER AND BABY	NERVOUS SYSTEM	REPRODUCTIVE SYSTEM	EAR, NOSE AND THROAT	URINARY SYSTEM	HERBS
Enhances immunity, antimicrobial.		Tiredness, lethargy.		Decongestant, colds, flu, catarrh.	Fluid retention, infections.	*Tropaolum majus* Nasturtium
Allergies.	Stimulates milk in nursing mothers.		Regulates periods.	Catarrh, asthma, hay fever.	Fluid retention.	*Urtica dioica* Stinging nettle
		Insomnia, anxiety, tension, headaches.	Period pain.			*Valeriana officinalis* Valerian
Earache, chest & throat infections.	Croup.	Neuralgia, head-aches, Anaesthetic.		Dry coughs, sore throat, bronchitis, catarrh, sinusitis, hay fever, asthma. Expectorant.	Fluid retention, cystitis.	*Verbascum thapsus* Mullein
	Enhances milk supply in nursing mothers. Avoid in pregnancy.	Anxiety, depression & stress-related symptoms. Tonic for nerves.	Regulates periods.		Fluid retention.	*Verbena officinalis* Vervain
			Heavy periods.	Catarrh, sore throats, chest problems.		*Vinca minor/ major* Lesser/ Greater periwinkle
Anti-inflammatory.				Harsh coughs, chest infections, catarrh.		*Viola odorata* Sweet violet
Anti-inflammatory.	Whooping cough & croup in babies.			Bronchitis, harsh coughs, catarrh, inflammatory chest problems, asthma. Expectorant.	Cystitis, fluid retention.	*Viola tricolor* Wild pansy

GLOSSARY

Alkaloids Naturally occurring chemical compounds that contain nitrogen. Common alkaloids are caffeine in coffee and nicotine in tobacco. Alkaloids may be toxic if taken in large amounts, and the medicinal use of some herbs that contain them is legally restricted to qualified doctors and herbalists.

Alterative Having a beneficial effect by aiding eliminative pathways throughout the body, thereby detoxifying the system.

Antibacterial Inhibits the growth of bacterial infections.

Antifungal Inhibits the growth of fungal infections.

Antihistamine Able to neutralize the effect of histamine (a chemical released by the body during allergic reactions) to treat allergies.

Antioxidant Reduces the damaging effect of free radicals which are involved in the onset of degenerative diseases such as heart disease and cancer, and in the ageing process.

Antiparasitic Inhibits the development of parasitic infestations.

Antiviral Inhibits the development of viral infections.

Bitters Bitter ingredients of herbs which enhance appetite and improve the digestion and absorption of food. Some bitter herbs also benefit the nervous and immune systems.

Cultivar Short for "cultivated variety" – a plant which has been constitently grown and kept under cultivation, rather than one which originated in the wild.

Demulcent A substance which is soothing to irritated tissues, especially mucous membranes.

Diuretic A substance which increases the flow of urine.

Emmenagogue A substance which promotes menstruation. Emmenagogues should be avoided during pregnancy.

Expectorant Promotes the expulsion of mucous from the respiratory tract.

Flavonoids Naturally-occurring chemical compounds which give an orange/yellow colour to plants such as cowslips. Some herbs containing flavonoids, such as burdock, tend to be diuretic in their action. Some, like liquorice, are anti-inflammatory.

Macerate To soak a substance, thereby softening it and allowing it to break down into its constituent parts.

Mucilage A gel-like substance that forms a viscous fluid when water is added to it. Mucilage has demulcent properties, and plants which contain it, such as flax, often make soothing laxatives.

Panacea A universal "cure-all" or remedy for all ailments.

Parturient Hastens and eases childbirth.

Saponins Naturally-occurring chemical compounds that form a soap-like lather when mixed with water. They have a variety of different therapeutic actions – they can be diuretic or expectorant. Steroidal saponins mimic precursors of female hormones.

Tannins Found in herbs such as agrimony and witch hazel, tannins have an astringent action, helping to prevent infections, to reduce inflammation and to speed healing. Herbs with a high tannin content make good compresses for cuts and wounds.

Volatile Oils Made up of many different chemical compounds, volatile oils are found in highly-scented herbs. All have antiseptic and antimicrobial actions, and some, such as chamomile, have anti-inflammatory and antispasmodic properties, while others, such as hyssop act as expectorants.

SEED COMPANIES & NURSERIES

Abundant Life Seed
Foundation
PO Box 772
Port Townsend, WA 98368
T: 206-385-5660

Agway, Inc. Seed Division
PO Box 4933
Syracuse, NY 13221

Bountiful Gardens
18001 Shafer Ranch Road
Willits, CA 96490
T: 707-459-6410

Bonanza Seed
International
PO Box V
Gilroy, CA 95020

Burgess Seed and Plant
Company
905 Four Seasons Road
Bloomington, IL 61701

W. Atlee Burpee & Co.
300 Park Avenue
Warminster, PA 18974
T: 215-674-4915

Companion Plants
PO Box 88
Athens, OH 47501
T: 614-592-4643

Caprilands Nursery
Silver Street
Coventry, CT 06238
T: 203-742-7244

Catnip Acres Farm
67 Christian Street
Oxford, CT 06483
T: 203-888-5649

The Cook's Garden
PO Box 535
Londonderry, VT 05148
T: 802-824-3400

Crockett Seed Company
PO Box 237
Metamora, OH 43540

Cruikshank's, Inc.
1015 Mount Pleasant Road
Toronto, Ontario, Canada
M4P 2M1
T: 416-488-8292

DeGiorgi Seed Co.
6011 N Street
Omaha, NE 68117
T: 402-731-3901

Earl May Seed & Nursey
Shenandoah, IA 51603

Gurney's Seed & Nursery
110 Capitol
Yankton, SD 57079
T: 605-665-1930

Harris Moran Seed Co.
60-A Saginaw Drive
Rochester, New York
14623
T: 716-442-6910

Harris Moran Seed Co.
1155 Harkins Road
Salinas, CA 93901

H.G. Hastings Company
1036 White Street SW
PO Box 115535
Atlanta, Georgia 30310
T: 404-755-6580

Henry Field's Seed and
Nursery Co.
415 N. Burnett Street
Shenandoah, IA 51602
T: 605-665-9391

Filaree Garlic Farm
Route 2, Box 162
Okanogan, Washington
98840-9774
T: 509-422-6940

Fox Hill Farm
440 W. Michigan Avenue
Parma, MI
T: 517-531-3179

The Gathered Herb
12114 N. State Road
Otisville, MI 48463
T: 313-631-6572

Glock's Herbs and Spices
2214 Sue Avenue
Orlando, FL 32803 (by
appt. only)
T: 407-898-5663

Hemlock Hill Herb Farm
Hemloch Hill Road
Litchfield, CT 06759-0415

High Altitude Gardens
PO Box 1048
Hailey, ID 83333

Hilltop Herb Farm
Ranch Road
PO Box 1734
Cleveland, TX 77327
T: 713-592-5859

Horticultural Enterprises
PO Box 810082
Dallas, TX 75381

J.L. Hudson, Seedsman
PO Box 1058
Redwood, CA 94064

Jackson & Perkins
1 Rose Lane
Medford, OR 97501
T: 503-776-2000

Johnny's Selected Seed
305 Foss Hill Road
Albion, Maine 04910
T: 207-437-4301

Jung Seeds and Nursery
335 S. High Street
Randolph, WI 53957
T: 414-326-3121

Le Jardin du Gourmet
PO Box 275G
St. Johnsbury Center,
Vermont 05863
T: 802-748-1446

Le Marche Seeds
International
PO Box 190
Dixon, CA 95620
T: 916-678-9244

Liberty Seed Company
PO Box 806
New Philadelphia, OH
44663
T: 216-364-1611

Logee's Greenhouses
141 North Street
Danielson, CT 06239
T: 203-774-8038

Meadowbrook Herb Farm
Route 138
Wyoming, RI
T: 401-539-7603

Mellinger's
2310 W. South Range
Street
North Lima, OH 44452
T: 216-549-9861

The Meyer Seed Co.
600 S. Carolina Street
Baltimore, MD 21231
T: 410-342-4224

Midwest Seed Growers
10559 Lackman Street
Lenexa, Kansas 66219
T; 913-894-0050

Native Seeds/SEARCH
2509 N. Campbell, #325
Tuscon, AZ 95719

Nichols Garden Surgery
1190 North Pacific
Highway
Albany, OR 97321
T: 503-928-9280

L.L. Olds Seed Co.
PO Box 1069
Madison, WI 53701
T: 608-249-9291

Park Seed Company
Cokesbury Road
Greenwood, SC 29467
T: 803-223-7333

Piedmont Plant Co.
PO Box 424
Albany, GA 31702
T: 912-883-7029

Pinetree Garden Seeds
PO Box 300
New Gloucester, ME
04260
T: 207-926-3400

Plants of the Southwest
Agua Fria Road
Route 6
PO Box 11A
Santa Fe, NM 87501

Redwood City Seed Co.
PO Box 361
Redwood City, CA 94064
T: 415-325-7333

Richter's
357 Highway 47
Goodwood, Ontario,
Canada LOC1AO
T: 416-640-6677

Rispens, Martin & Sons
3332 Ridge Road
Lansing, IL 60438
T: 708-474-0241

Roswell Seed Company
115-177 South Main Street
Roswell, NM 88201
T: 505-622-7701

Sandy Mush Herb Nursery
316 Surrett Cove Road
Leicester, NC 28748
T: 704-683-2014

Seeds Blum
Idaho City Stage
Boise, ID 83706
T: 208-342-0858

Seeds of Change
621 Old Sante Fe Trail
Suite 10
Santa Fe, NM 88038
T: 505-983-8956

Seed Savers Exchange
Box 239
Decorah, IA 52101

Shepherd's Garden Seeds
7389 West Zayante Road
Felton, CA 95018
T: 408-335-5400
30 Irene street
Torrington, CT 06790

Southern Exposure Seed
Exchange
PO Box 158
North Garden, VA 22959
T: 804-973-4703

Sunnybrook Herb Farm
Box 6
Chesterland, OH 44026
T: 216-729-7232

Talavaya Seeds
PO Box 707
Santa Cruz Station
Santa Cruz, NM 87507

Taylor's Herb Gardens
1535 Lone Oad Road
Vista, CA 92084
T: 619-717-3485

Territorial Seed Co.
PO Box 157
Cottage Grove, OR 97424
T: 503-942-9547

Thompson & Morgan
PO Box 1308
Jackson, NY 08527
T: 201-363-2225

Twilley Seeds
PO Box 65
Trevose, PA 19053

Well-Sweep Herb Farm
317 Mt. Bethel Road
Port Murray, NJ 07865

Wyatt-Quarles Seed Co.
PO Box 739
Garner, NC 27529
T: 219-772-4243

INDEX

Page numbers in **bold** indicate illustrated main entries; those followed by *p* (*passim*) indicate that
there are scattered references to that topic within those pages.

A

abrasions 45, 55, 118, 120
abscesses 60, 121, 123
absorption 46, 55, 57, 59, 89, 108
acne 62, 67, 77, 99, 114, 117, 120, 121
ageing 46, 87, 104
agrimony 20, 24, 34, **113**, 126-7
AIDS 62
alcoholism 86, 101
American angelica 50
American vervain 109
anaemia 46, 89, 95, 120
anaesthetics 60
analgesics 64
angelica 14-18*p*, 20, 22-5*p*, 28, 29, **49-50**, 128-9
angina 115
anti-allergenics 62, 68
antibacterials 45, 46, 49, 57, 58, 60, 73, 74, 95, 114
antibiotics 81, 93, 114
antidepressants, withdrawal from 54, 100
  see also depression
antifungals 45, 46, 54, 57, 62, 74, 95, 114
antihistamines 57, 103
anti-inflammatories 44, 45, 57, 58, 62, 64, 68, 81,
  83, 90, 93, 99, 103, 110, 111, 114, 117, 121, 123
antimalarials 53, 71
antimicrobials 73, 87, 94, 105
antioxidants 46, 87, 104
antiparasitics 45
antiseptics 44, 46, 51, 53, 54, 57, 64, 74, 77, 82,
  83, 85, 89, 103, 104, 116
antispasmodics 66, 81
anti-tumour activity 55, 56, 110
antivirals 45, 46, 60, 73
appetite 51, 53, 56, 57, 59, 60, 76, 83, 89, 95, 105,
  108, 114, 124
apple trees, companion herbs for 27
aromatherapy, herbs for 24
aromatic gardens 22-4, 25
arrhythmia 115
arteriosclerosis 60, 111
arthritis 51, 57-9*p*, 62-4*p*, 68, 71, 76, 81, 86, 87,
  89, 90, 94, 95, 98-101*p*, 103, 108, 110, 111, 113,
  114, 116, 117, 120-4*p*
asparagus, companion herbs for 27
asthma 46, 48-50*p*, 57, 58, 68, 71, 73, 74, 81,
  84-6*p*, 88, 89, 97, 98, 103, 104, 106, 111, 123,
  124
astringents 44, 45, 54, 76, 90, 94, 101, 109, 113,
  120, 124
atherosclerosis 64, 115

B

babies 56, 66-7*p*, 84
  see also nursing mothers
basil 14, 17, 20, 21, 24, 26-9*p*, 34, **85**, 138-9
baths, herbal 40
bay, sweet 14, 17, 20, 28, 31, **76-7**, 136-7
beans, companion herbs for 27
beauty aids 45

bergamot 31
Bethlehem sage 92
bistort 17, 20, 24, **89-90**, 140-1
bites 48, 58, 69, 85
black cohosh 15, 17, 23, 58, 130-1
blood 44, 46, 54, 58, 78, 81, 86, 88, 105, 106, 108,
  111, 114, 115, 121, 122
  bleeding 55, 66, 69, 90, 92, 94, 101, 109,
    120, 124
blue vervain 109
body system thematic garden groupings 20
boils 60, 99, 117, 121, 123
bone repair 102
boneset (herb) 63
borage 17, 23, 26-9*p*
bowels 45, 51, 54, 72, 77, 83, 84, 104, 106, 114
breast milk *see* nursing mothers
breast pain 58
bronchitis 48, 58, 74, 76, 81, 84, 92, 95, 106, 111,
  123
bruises 69, 72, 85
brussel sprouts, companion herbs for 27
burdock 14, 16, 20, 24, 29, 34, **113-14**, 128-9
burns 44, 48, 55, 57, 69, 72, 77, 85, 92, 94, 95,
  102, 120-4*p*

C

cabbages, companion herbs for 27
cancers 54, 56, 110
candida/candidiasis *see* thrush
capsules 39
caraway thyme 104
carrots
  companion herbs for 27
  wild carrot 14, 20, 24, **116**, 132-3
catarrh 44, 45, 49, 50, 53, 56, 69, 73, 74, 76, 79,
  83, 85, 90, 92, 93, 98, 101, 103, 104, 109, 111,
  114, 118, 124
catmint/catnip 14, 16, 25, **84-5**, 138-9
cauliflowers, companion herbs for 27
celandines 17
celery
  companion herbs for 27
  wild celery **50-1**, 128-9
cell production 102
cellulite 66
chamomile 14, 16-18*p*, 20-9*p*, 31, 32, 34, **56-7**
  cream 41
chest 60, 68, 73, 74, 76, 77, 81, 84, 87, 88, 92-7*p*,
  104, 106, 109-11*p*, 118
chicken pox 44, 64, 84, 98, 117
chickweed 20, 24, **122-3**, 144-5
chicory **57-8**, 130-1
childbirth 45, 49, 51, 53, 57-9*p*, 69, 76, 78, 83,
  89, 94-5, 97
  see also pregnancy, herbs to avoid during
Chinese angelica 50
Chinese motherwort 78
chives 14-18*p*, 21, 23, 26-8*p*, 34, 46, 126-7
cholesterol 46, 54, 60, 68, 81, 86
cilantro *see* coriander/cilantro

circulation 44, 46, 50, 56, 62, 73, 74, 76, 78, 79,
  83, 84, 87, 89, 94, 98, 105, 111, 114, 115, 121, 122
cirrhosis 101
clary sage 16, 17, 20, 24, 25, **97-8**, 142-3
cleavers/clivers 20, 24, **116-17**, 134-5
colds 34, 44, 45, 49, 53, 60, 71, 73, 74, 76, 77, 84,
  85, 87, 90, 93-5*p*, 98, 103, 104, 114, 118, 122
cold sores 55
colic 48-50*p*, 56, 58, 59, 64, 66, 72, 73, 76, 83, 84,
  88, 89, 95, 97, 101, 106, 116, 122
colitis 44, 45, 48, 69, 81, 83, 90, 113, 123
comfrey 14, 16, 17, 20, 23, 24, 26, 28, 31, 35, **102**,
  144-5
common skullcap *see* skullcaps
companion planting 26, 27, 45, 46, 51, 53, 54, 73
compost heap 26
compresses 41
cone flower *see* purple cone flower
conjunctivitis 59, 120
constipation 49, 54, 57, 66, 73, 85, 99, 108, 120
containers, herbs in 26-8
coriander/cilantro 14, 16, 17, 20, 21, 23, 24, 26-9*p*,
  31, 59, 130-1
Corsican mint 29
coughs 45, 46, 48-50*p*, 68, 71, 76, 81, 84, 85, 88,
  90, 92, 97, 98, 104, 106, 109-11*p*, 114
courgettes, companion herbs for 27
cowslip 15, 16, 20, 25, **90-1**, 140-1
cradle cap 67
cramp 58, 85, 88
creams, herbal 40-1
Crohn's disease 83
croup 48, 81, 88, 106, 111
cucumbers, companion herbs for 27
curled dock *see* dock
cuts 44, 45, 55, 72, 85, 92, 95, 102, 109, 118, 120,
  124
cuttings, propagation by 31-2
cystitis 45, 48, 51, 59, 62, 76, 81, 104, 108, 111, 116,
  117, 120

D

dandelion 20, 24, 26, 34, **123-4**, 144-5
debility 120
decoctions 36, 39-40
decongestants 45, 73, 76, 77, 84, 85, 87, 90, 98,
  103, 105, 106, 109, 110, 114
depression 49, 51, 54, 72, 77, 82, 85, 87, 89, 90,
  94, 97, 100, 108, 122
  see also antidepressants, withdrawl from
detoxicants 51, 53-5*p*, 62, 64, 67, 73, 77, 79, 81,
  89, 93, 95, 98, 99, 101, 103-5*p*, 111, 114,
  116-18*p*, 120, 121, 124
diabetes 54, 58, 109, 110, 114
diarrhoea 44, 45, 49, 55, 56, 64, 66, 69, 83, 84,
  90, 94, 101, 104, 109, 113, 120, 122
digestion 44, 46, 48-51*p*, 53, 55-7*p*, 59, 60,
  64, 67-8*p*, 71, 73, 74, 79, 81, 83, 86, 89, 93-7*p*,
  100, 101, 103-5*p*, 108, 109, 113-18*p*, 120,
  122-4*p*
dill 14, 16, 17, 20, 21, 26-9*p*, 31, 34, 49, 128-9

diuretics 45, 48, 51, 58, 60, 62-4*p*, 66, 67, 71, 78, 79, 81, 82, 87, 89, 94, 95, 98, 101, 104, 105, 108, 111, 113-18*p*, 120-4*p*
diverticulitis 72
dock 20, 24, **120-1**, 142-3
drying herbs 34-5
dysentry 69, 90, 109

E

ears 49, 108
echinacea *see* purple cone flower
eczema 44, 57, 67, 83, 86, 99, 117, 120, 123, 124
elder 20, 22, 24, 28, 34, **98**, 142-3
elecampane 14, 16, 17, 20, 23, 31, 34, **74**, 136-7
enteritis 55, 64, 81, 104
epilepsy 100
essential oils 40, 41-2
evening primrose 22, 25, 29, **86**, 138-9
expectorants 45, 68, 73, 74, 76, 81, 82, 84, 90, 92, 99, 106, 111, 114, 117
eyes 39, 49, 59, 64, 66, 69, 97, 98, 113, 118, 120

F

facial scrubs 54
fallopian tube infection 104
fennel 14-17*p*, 20, 21, 23-6*p*, 29, 31, 34, 59, 64, 66, 132-3
feverfew 26, 28, **102-3**, 144-5
fevers 44, 50, 53, 55, 56, 59, 63, 64, 66, 73, 74, 79, 83, 84, 87, 90, 93-5*p*, 98, 100, 101, 103, 104, 108, 110, 111, 114, 117, 118
fibroids 45
figwort 20, 24, **121-2**, 142-3
flax/linseed 20, **79-81**, 136-7
Florence fennel 64
flu 44, 53, 54, 57, 60, 73, 77, 81, 84, 85, 87, 90, 93-5*p*, 98, 104, 114, 118
fluid retention *see* diuretics
food poisoning 53
freezing herbs 35
fruits, companion planting with 27
fumitory 20, 24, **67**, 134-5
fungal infections *see* antifungals

G

gall bladder 57, 59, 94, 105, 113, 122, 124
gallstones 58
gargles 39, 45, 48, 66, 90, 94, 104, 109, 113, 118, 120
garlic 20, 27, 28, **45-6**, 126-7
gastritis 44, 45, 48, 59, 64, 76, 81, 113, 123
gastro-enteritis 45, 104, 120
genito-urinary infections 45, 76, 104
gentian 17
German chamomile *see* chamomile
glandular fever 60
globe artichoke 16, 23, **59-60**, 132-3
goldenrod 34, 101, 144-5
gout 51, 57, 62, 63, 66, 71, 87, 89, 90, 95, 98, 99, 101, 111, 114, 116, 117, 120-4*p*
grapes, companion herbs for 27
gravel 45, 63, 64, 115, 116
greater periwinkle 20, 32, **109-10**, 146-7
greater plantain 20, 24, **118**, 140-1
gripe water 49, 66

ground ivy 17, 20, 24, 34, **117-18**, 134-5
gums 48, 66, 90, 94, 120

H

haemorrhoids 44, 69, 90, 92, 109, 120
harvesting herb plants 34
hawthorn 20, 24, 31, **115**, 130-1
hay fever 45, 57, 83, 103, 108, 114, 124
headache 49, 56-8*p*, 64, 76, 77, 81, 82, 85, 87-90*p*, 94, 97, 100, 103, 106-8*p*, 118, 120, 122
healing properties, thematic garden grouping according to 20
heart 46, 54, 58, 78, 106, 115
heartburn 48, 60, 66, 68, 83
heather 15, 16, 20, **62**, 132-3
heavy metals, removing 81
hemp agrimony 63
hepatitis 101
herbaceous borders, herbs in 16-18
herb gardens 14-32
herpes 54, 74, 84, 87
HIV treatments 62, 73
Hodgkin's disease 76, 110
hollyhock 15
holy thistle **55-6**, 130-1
honeysuckle *see* wild honeysuckle
hops 20, 23-5*p*, **71-2**, 134-5
horehound 20
hormone regulation 54, 86
horseradish 16, 20, 24, 27, 28, **114-15**, 128-9
hot flushes *see* menopause
hyperactivity 56-7, 86
hyssop 14, 16-27*p*, 29, 34, **73**, 136-7

I

immune system 45, 46, 53, 54, 56, 60, 63, 73, 86, 93, 94, 103
indigestion 44, 49, 50, 56, 66, 68, 72, 76, 77, 83-5*p*, 89, 97, 108, 116, 122, 124
infusions 36-7, 39-40
insect bites 48, 69
insect repellents 26, 28, 77, 117
insomnia 49, 57, 62, 71, 77, 82, 87, 88, 90, 97, 106, 108, 115
iris 25
irritability 49, 57, 58, 108
irritable bladder 48, 81, 89
irritable bowel 72, 104, 106

J

jasmine 20, 23-5*p*, **74**, 76, 136-7
jaundice 60, 101
jet lag 72
Joe Pye weed 20, **63**, 132-3
juniper 14, 16, 17, 20

K

kidneys 63, 64, 79, 81, 89, 121, 124
knot gardens 18, 19

L

lady's mantle 14, 16, 20, 31, **44-5**, 126-7
lavender 14, 16, 17, 19-26*p*, 28, 29, 32, **77-8**, 136-7

laxatives 67, 81, 99, 110, 114, 120, 121
leeks 27
lemon balm 14, 17, 18, 20-5*p*, 28, 34, 35, **82-3**, 138-9
lemon-scented thyme 104
lesser periwinkle *see* periwinkles
lesser plantain *see* plantains
lesser skullcap *see* skullcaps
lethargy 56, 84, 105, 122
lettuces, companion herbs for 27
leukaemia 110
liniments 42
linseed/flax 20, 27, 28, **79-81**, 136-7
liquorice **68-9**, 134-5
liver 51, 53, 55-7*p*, 59, 60, 66-8*p*, 74, 86, 94, 95, 99, 101, 103-5*p*, 108, 113, 114, 117, 120, 122, 124
lovage 14-17*p*, 20, 23, 28, **79**, 136-7
lungwort 14, 17, 20, 21, 24, **92**, 140-1
lymphatic system 55, 76, 117, 120, 121

M

Madagascan periwinkle 110
malaria 53, 71
marigold 15-18*p*, 20, 21, 25-7*p*, 29, 31, **54-5**, 130-1
marjoram 14, 16-18*p*, 20, 21, 23, 24, 27, 28, 35, **87**, 138-9
marsh mallow 14, 16, 17, 20, 24, 46, 48, **126-7**
mastitis 121
meadow sage 98
meadowsweet 14-17*p*, 20, 23-5*p*, 64, 132-3
measles 44, 60, 64, 84, 98, 114, 117
medicine wheels in physic garden 21
menopause 55, 58, 66, 68, 72, 78, 86, 95, 97, 115
menstrual cycle 44, 45, 48-51*p*, 53, 55-7*p*, 59, 63, 66, 69, 76, 78, 79, 83, 84, 86-8*p*, 90, 93-5*p*, 97, 100, 101, 104, 106, 108, 109, 124
migraine 77, 86, 89, 94, 103
milk thistle 16, 23, **100-1**, 144-5
mints 14, 17, 20-3*p*, 27-9*p*, 34, 35
motherwort 14, 20, 31, **78**, 136-7
mouse repellents 28
mouth ulcers 90, 103, 120
mouthwashes 66, 94, 120
mugwort 53
mullein 15-17*p*, 20, 24, 29, 34, **106-8**, 146-7
mumps 60
muscles 48, 49, 58, 62, 69, 71, 77, 84, 85, 87, 88, 90, 104, 106
myrtle 17

N

nasturtium 17, 18, 27, 28, **104-5**, 146-7
nausea 49, 50, 60, 66, 77, 83, 85, 101
nervous exhaustion 49, 54, 106
nettle, stinging 20, 24, 26, **124-5**, 146-7
spray 28
stings 121
nettle rash (urticaria) 123
neuralgia 49, 57, 58, 64, 82, 88, 108
night sweats *see* menopause
North American wild strawberry 67
nursing mothers 49, 56, 66, 89, 95, 99, 108, 117, 124
    see also babies

O

oestrogen 54, 58, 68, 95
onions 27
oregano 25, 29

P

palpitations 77, 78, 100, 115
pancreas 105
pansy, wild 20, 24, 111, 146-7
Parkinson's disease 88
parsley 14, 16-18*p*, 20, 21, 23, 26-8*p*, 34, 35, 88-9, 140-1
parsley piert 45
parsnips, companion herbs for 27
pasque flower 14, 16, 20, 23, 24, 48-9, 128-9
passionflower 87-8, 138-9
patios, herbs on 28, 29
pelvic inflammatory disease 45, 62, 63, 93
pennyroyal 16, 17, 23, 25, 28, 29
peppermint 14, 20, 83-4, 138-9
peptic ulcers 56, 59, 113
periods *see* menstrual cycle
periwinkles 20, 32, 109-10, 146-7
phlebitis 69
physic gardens 19-22
piles 123, 124
plantains 20, 24, 118, 140-1
pleurisy 73, 123
PMS 50, 83, 86, 87
post-natal depression 97
potatoes, companion herbs for 27
pot herbs, buying 29-30
poultices 41, 48
pregnancy, herbs to avoid during 45, 51, 53, 55, 58, 78, 79, 89, 97, 103, 116
   see also childbirth
propagation methods for herbs 29-32
prostate gland 62, 63, 116
psoriasis 67, 99, 114, 117, 120
psyllium *see* plantains
purple cone flower (echinacea) 15, 17, 20, 23, 60-2, 132-3

R

radishes, companion herbs for 27
rashes 45, 48, 64, 84, 93, 98, 121, 123
raspberry 94-5, 142-3
rattlesnake bites 58
relaxants 48, 49, 56, 71, 76, 78, 82, 83, 85, 86, 88, 90, 93, 97, 98, 100, 115
remedies, preparation of 36-42
restoratives *see* tonics
rheumatism 51, 58, 64, 71, 76, 81, 94, 99, 108, 123
ribwort plantain *see* plantains
Roman chamomile *see* chamomile
root division, propagation by 31
rose 20, 22-5*p*, 92-3, 140-1
rosemary 14, 17-22*p*, 24, 25, 27-9*p*, 31, 34, 93-4, 140-1
roundworms 51
rue 14, 16, 28
Russian comfrey 102

S

sage 14, 15, 17, 18, 20-3*p*, 25, 27, 29, 32, 34, 95-7, 142-3
St John's wort 20, 23, 24, 34, 72-3, 134-5
salpingitis 76
salves 40
scabies 74
scalds 48, 57, 77, 85, 92, 94, 102, 121, 123-4*p*
sciatica 103, 122
seasonal affective disorder (SAD) 72
seed, wild herbs from 24, 29, 30-1
sex 79, 87, 93
shingles 88, 103
sinusitis 106, 114
skin 44, 45, 48, 53, 54, 57-9*p*, 62, 67, 69, 74, 77, 81, 86, 90, 93, 98, 99, 109, 111, 114, 117, 120-4*p*
skullcaps 14, 20, 23, 34, 99-100, 142-3
soapwort 14, 16, 99, 142-3
soil types and herb planting 14
sores 55, 57, 72, 92, 95, 102, 121
sore throat *see* throat
southernwood 16-18*p*, 24-7*p*, 31, 51-3, 128-9
spastic colon 104
splinters, drawing out 48
sprains 69, 72
steroid treatment, withdrawal from 68
stinging nettle *see* nettle, stinging
stings 85, 121
stones 45, 63, 64, 101, 109, 115, 116
storing herbs 35
strawberries 27, 28
   wild strawberry 17, 20, 23, 24, 28, 66-7, 132-3
stress 56, 59, 68, 72, 76-8*p*, 81, 82, 84, 85, 87, 88, 90, 97, 100, 106, 108, 115
sunburn 48, 72, 95, 98, 120, 123
sunflower 69-71, 134-5
suppositories 39
sweet bay *see* bay
sweet fennel *see* fennel
sweet marjoram *see* marjoram
sweet violet *see* violet
sweet woodruff 117
sweet wormwood 53
syrups 37-8

T

tablets 39
tansy 28
tarragon 23
thematic plant grouping in garden 20
threadworms 51
throat 45, 48, 59, 60, 66, 71, 77, 81, 85, 87, 90, 93-5*p*, 98, 104, 106, 109, 113, 118, 120, 123
thrombosis 81
thrush 54, 57, 104, 114
thyme 14-18*p*, 20-3*p*, 25-9*p*, 32, 34, 103-4, 144-5
tinctures 38, 40
tissue repair 44, 77
tomatoes, companion herbs for 27
tonics 46, 48, 50, 51, 54, 55, 67, 73, 85, 89, 90, 93, 94, 97, 100, 106, 108, 114, 122, 124
tonsilitis 121
toothache 57
tormentil 20, 24, 118, 120, 140-1
tranquillisers, withdrawal from 54, 100
travel sickness 83, 101

triglyceride levels 60
tuberculosis 74, 95
tumours 56, 110

U

ulcers 44, 55, 64, 68, 72, 77, 90, 92, 94, 95, 101-3*p*, 120-3*p*
   peptic 56, 59, 113
   varicose 69, 90, 123
urethritis 62
urinary system 45, 51, 60, 62-4*p*, 66, 101, 104, 105, 109, 113-17*p*, 120, 124
urticaria 123
uterus 58, 69, 78, 94-5, 97

V

vaginal infections 45, 54, 57, 104, 114
valerian 14, 16, 17, 20, 31, 34, 105-6, 146-7
varicose veins 44, 69, 72, 90, 92, 109
vegetable garden, herbs in 26-7
vervain 20, 108-9, 146-7
violet, sweet 14-17*p*, 24, 25, 110, 146-7
Virginian skullcap *see* skullcaps
vomiting 83

W

warts 124
whooping cough 58, 81, 104, 111
wild carrot 14, 20, 24, 116, 132-3
wild celery 50-1, 128-9
wild herb gardens 24-6
wild honeysuckle 23-5*p*, 81-2, 138-9
wild oats 20, 54, 130-1
wild pansy 20, 24, 111, 146-7
wild strawberry 17, 20, 23, 24, 28, 66-7, 132-3
wild thyme 104
wind 44, 49, 50, 56, 64, 66, 76, 77, 83, 84, 89, 104, 122
witch hazel 20, 32, 34, 69, 134-5
wood betony 20, 24, 122, 144-5
woodruff, sweet 117
worms 51, 53, 55, 74, 116
wormwood 14-17*p*, 19, 20, 22, 25-9*p*, 53, 128-9
wounds 44, 45, 55, 72, 74, 85, 92, 95, 101, 102, 104, 109, 118, 120, 121, 124

Y

yarrow 16, 20, 23-5*p*, 25, 28, 29, 31, 34, 44, 126-7
yellow dock *see* dock

Z

zucchini, companion herbs for 27

Edited by Laura Wilson
Editorial Assistance by Elizabeth Haylett
Photography by Juliette Wade
Illustrations by Madeline David

Additional Photography:

A-Z Botanical Collection pp.58, 67C, 68, 80, 88L, 120
David Armstrong pp.1, 30, 32, 35-9, 40-2, 46R, 55L, 56L,
62, 66, 69, 77, 82, 85, 88R, 110
Nigel Bradley pp.48L, 60, 103
The photographs which appear on the following pages
were taken in the author's garden:

pp.6, 9, 11, 48L, 52, 57, 61, 65, 70, 72, 75, 79, 84, 86, 89, 91, 92, 95,
97, 99, 100, 103, 104, 105, 107, 109, 111, 112,
113, 116, 119, 123L, 125, endpapers

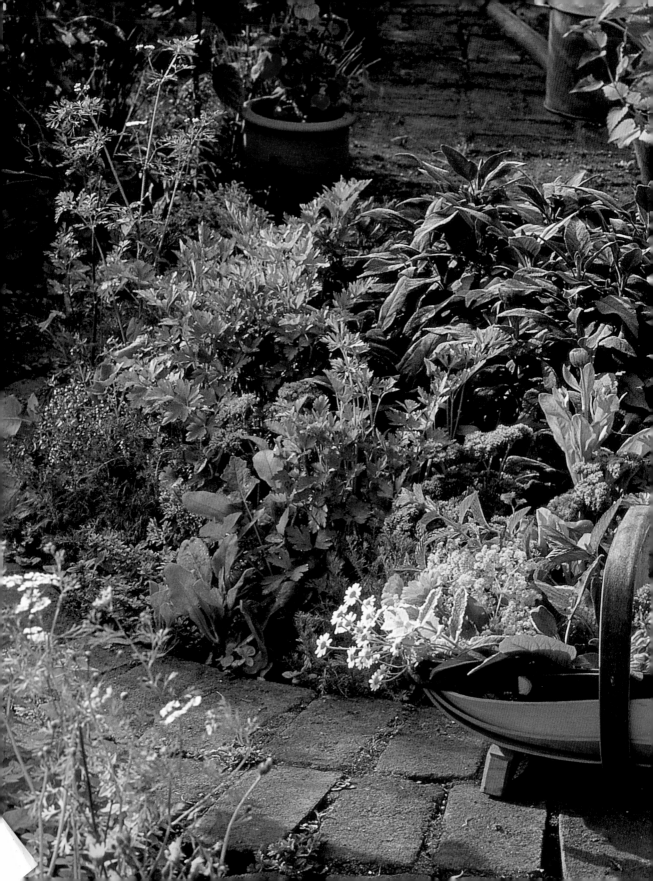

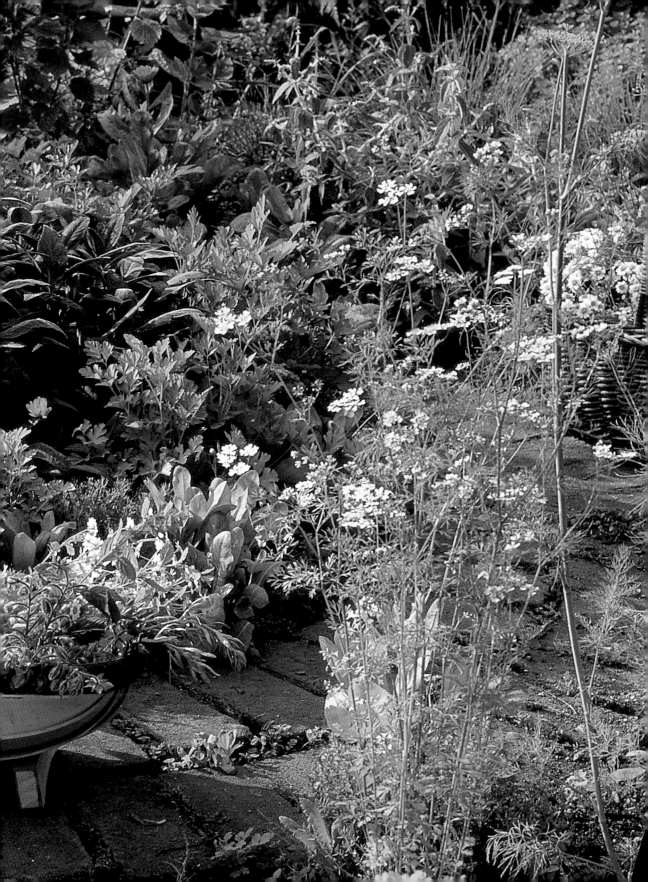